Measurement Technologies for up- and Downstream Bioprocessing

Measurement Technologies for up- and Downstream Bioprocessing

Editor

Carl-Fredrik Mandenius

MDPI • Basel • Beijing • Wuhan • Barcelona • Belgrade • Manchester • Tokyo • Cluj • Tianjin

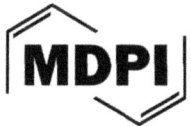

Editor
Carl-Fredrik Mandenius
Division of Biotechnology, IFM,
Linkoping University
Sweden

Editorial Office
MDPI
St. Alban-Anlage 66
4052 Basel, Switzerland

This is a reprint of articles from the Special Issue published online in the open access journal *Processes* (ISSN 2227-9717) (available at: https://www.mdpi.com/journal/processes/special_issues/measurement_technology_bioprocessing).

For citation purposes, cite each article independently as indicated on the article page online and as indicated below:

LastName, A.A.; LastName, B.B.; LastName, C.C. Article Title. *Journal Name* **Year**, *Volume Number*, Page Range.

ISBN 978-3-0365-1150-4 (Hbk)
ISBN 978-3-0365-1151-1 (PDF)

Cover image courtesy of Carl-Fredrik Mandenius.

© 2021 by the authors. Articles in this book are Open Access and distributed under the Creative Commons Attribution (CC BY) license, which allows users to download, copy and build upon published articles, as long as the author and publisher are properly credited, which ensures maximum dissemination and a wider impact of our publications.
The book as a whole is distributed by MDPI under the terms and conditions of the Creative Commons license CC BY-NC-ND.

Contents

About the Editor vii

Preface to "Measurement Technologies for up- and Downstream Bioprocessing" ix

Carl-Fredrik Mandenius
Measurement Technologies for Upstream and Downstream Bioprocessing
Reprinted from: *Processes* **2021**, *9*, 143, doi:10.3390/pr9010143 1

Lorenz Theuer, Judit Randek, Stefan Junne, Peter Neubauer, Carl-Fredrik Mandenius and Valerio Beni
Single-Use Printed Biosensor for L-Lactate and Its Application in Bioprocess Monitoring
Reprinted from: *Processes* **2020**, *8*, 321, doi:10.3390/pr8030321 5

Philipp Doppler, Lukas Veiter, Oliver Spadiut, Christoph Herwig and Vignesh Rajamanickam
A Chemometric Tool to Monitor and Predict Cell Viability in Filamentous Fungi Bioprocesses Using UV Chromatogram Fingerprints
Reprinted from: *Processes* **2020**, *8*, 461, doi:10.3390/pr8040461 23

Daniel A.M. Pais, Paulo R.S. Galrão, Anastasiya Kryzhanska, Jérémie Barbau, Inês A. Isidro and Paula M. Alves
Holographic Imaging of Insect Cell Cultures: Online Non-Invasive Monitoring of Adeno-Associated Virus Production and Cell Concentration
Reprinted from: *Processes* **2020**, *8*, 487, doi:10.3390/pr8040487 39

Christian Klinger, Verena Trinkaus and Tobias Wallocha
Novel Carbon Dioxide-Based Method for Accurate Determination of pH and pCO_2 in Mammalian Cell Culture Processes
Reprinted from: *Processes* **2020**, *8*, 520, doi:10.3390/pr8050520 55

Alexandra Hofer, Paul Kroll, Matthias Barmettler and Christoph Herwig
A Reliable Automated Sampling System for On-Line and Real-Time Monitoring of CHO Cultures
Reprinted from: *Processes* **2020**, *8*, 637, doi:10.3390/pr8060637 71

Stephen Goldrick, Alexandra Umprecht, Alison Tang, Roman Zakrzewski, Matthew Cheeks, Richard Turner, Aled Charles, Karolina Les, Martyn Hulley, Chris Spencer and Suzanne S. Farid
High-Throughput Raman Spectroscopy Combined with Innovate Data Analysis Workflow to Enhance Biopharmaceutical Process Development
Reprinted from: *Processes* **2020**, *8*, 1179, doi:10.3390/pr8091179 87

Thuy Tran, Olof Eskilson, Florian Mayer, Robert Gustavsson, Robert Selegård, Ingemar Lundström, Carl-Fredrik Mandenius, Erik Martinsson and Daniel Aili
Real-Time Nanoplasmonic Sensor for IgG Monitoring in Bioproduction
Reprinted from: *Processes* **2020**, *8*, 1302, doi:10.3390/pr8101302 119

Daniel A.M. Pais, Chris Brown, Anastasia Neuman, Krishanu Mathur, Inês A. Isidro, Paula M. Alves and Peter G. Slade
Dielectric Spectroscopy to Improve the Production of rAAV Used in Gene Therapy
Reprinted from: *Processes* **2020**, *8*, 1456, doi:10.3390/pr8111456 131

About the Editor

Carl-Fredrik Mandenius has been a professor in engineering biology at the Division of Biotechnology, Linköping University, Sweden, since 2000. He has previously worked in the pharmaceutical industry as director of PR&D and has been an associate professor at Lund University. His background is in biosensor technology and design and in bioprocess development, especially process measurement and control. He has been involved in several EU projects on biosensors, bioprocess monitoring and control, and new stem cell in vitro testing methodology using stem cell-derived organ cells.

Preface to "Measurement Technologies for up- and Downstream Bioprocessing"

This book is devoted to new developments in measurement technologies for upstream and downstream bioprocessing. The recent advances in biotechnology and bioprocessing have generated a number of new biological products that require more qualified analytical technologies for diverse process analytical needs. These include especially fast and sensitive measurement technology that, early in the process train, can inform on critical process parameters related to process economy and product quality and that can facilitate ambitions of designing efficient integrated end-to-end bioprocesses. This book covers these topics as well as analytical monitoring methods based either on real-time or in-line sensor technology, on simple and compact bioanalytical devices, or on the use of advanced data prediction methods.

The editor is most grateful to all of the authors for their contributions to the book and to the staff of MDPI for their excellent support.

Carl-Fredrik Mandenius
Editor

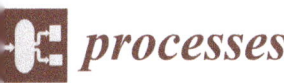

Editorial

Measurement Technologies for Upstream and Downstream Bioprocessing

Carl-Fredrik Mandenius

Department of Physics, Chemistry and Biology, Linköping University, 581 83 Linköping, Sweden; carl-fredrik.mandenius@liu.se

This special issue is devoted to new developments in measurement technologies for upstream and downstream bioprocessing. The recent advances in biotechnology and bioprocessing have generated a number of new biological products that require more qualified analytical technologies for diverse process analytical needs. This includes especially fast and sensitive measurement technology that early in the process train can inform on critical process parameters related to process economy and product quality and that can facilitate ambitions of designing efficient integrated end-to-end bioprocesses [1–3]. The flow of information about critical parameters should allow enhancement of productivity and better utilization of materials between process stages and unit operations. In integrated processes such information flows need to be faster than in conventional processes in order to allow the intended continuity (Figure 1). This is possible only with analytical monitoring methods based either on real-time or in-line sensor technology, on simple and compact bioanalytical devices, or use of advanced data prediction methods [4–7].

Although the Process Analytical Technology initiative, originally outlined by the pharmaceutical regulatory agencies, aims for pharmaceutical products, its relevance to bioprocess engineering is wider [8]. It may comprise all kinds of bioprocesses, from productions of small molecules, proteins, or cells for food and drugs, as well as commodity products. The aspects of quality-by-design, defining the design and control space for critical quality and process parameters are relevant beyond pharmaceutical processes. Industry, however, must achieve this quality within such economical frames that the production cost can cover. If quality cannot be achieved at a cost which is within the actual market value including coverage of upfront costs, sustainability of the product is lost. This calls for measurement technology which ensures both quality criteria and manufacturing efficiency.

The eight research articles in this special issue present novel approaches for advancing monitoring and control technology in these directions.

One angle of approach is about advancing the measurement principle itself to enhance sensitivity and selectivity when analysing critical parameters and attributes of cells and biomolecules, including viruses, proteins, and metabolites during bioprocessing.

This is successfully done with online digital holographic microscopy when monitoring a bioreactor culture with baculovirus-infected insect cells (Sf9 cells) that produce a recombinant adeno-associated virus. The digital holographic microscopy has the capacity to resolve in real time from samples withdrawn culture such important features as the viability of the insect cells and the titre of the produced virus [9]. With this information generated prior to subsequent downstream processing, efficient process integration can be expected.

Another novel measurement principle presented is nano-plasmonic sensing. This novel fibre-optical sensor technology allows rapid measurements of antibody (IgG) titres in bioprocesses [10]. The sensor is based on a combination of the optical effect of localized surface plasmon resonance with robust single-use Protein A-modified sensor chips to detect IgG molecules. The chip is housed in a flexible flow cell close to the process. This in-line technology has the capacity to be tailored to detect a variety of product molecules and their variants, either at early upstream stage or in later downstream stages for adaptation of the stages of benefit for integrated bioprocesses.

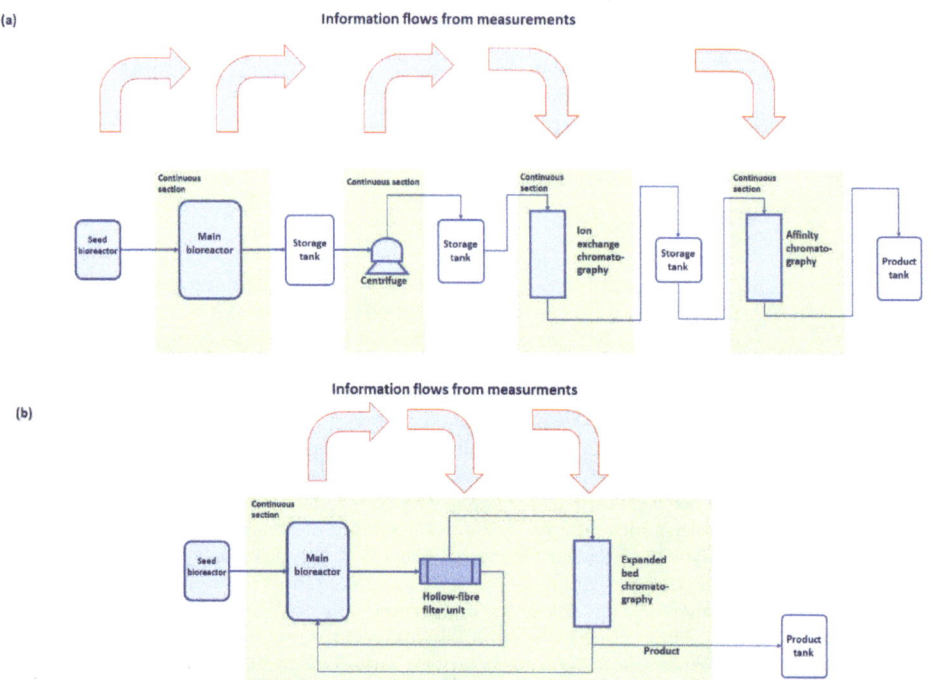

Figure 1. Bioprocess integration requires measurement technology that allows continuity and just-in-time information flow. (**a**) A conventional bioprocess with separate unit operations, (**b**) an end-to-end bioprocess with integrated and recycled flows between units. Depicted unit operations are examples.

Spectroscopic measurement technology can be developed further for at-line applications with the help of better spectral analysis methods to predict requirements in forthcoming stages. An example of this is high-throughput Raman spectroscopy microscopy using a spectral data analysis workflow to replace off-line analytics [11]. Promising results are shown for upstream applications with two mammalian cell lines that express different therapeutic proteins and demonstrate at-line monitoring of a high-throughput micro-bioreactor setup. This paves the way for improving process development and operation.

Another example of using established sensor technology for solving urgent bioanalytical needs is presented with in-line dielectric spectroscopy. Again, an insect cell-baculovirus expression vector system for large scale recombinant adeno-associated virus production is used, where the dielectric spectroscopy continuously monitors the production of the recombinant virus in the bioreactor [12]. As critically important when producing virus in insect cells, the cell concentration is monitored, and the infection time and cell viability at harvest are estimated with the purpose to enhance virus productivity and product quality. The use of in-line dielectric spectroscopy opens up for improving the robustness and control of the virus production.

A third example of exploiting an established methodology with smart computations is shown with size exclusion chromatography. Critical information on the release of impurity in *Penicillium chrysogenum* culture is captured from advanced data analysis [13]. The information is found in the ultraviolet chromatograms through fingerprinting principal component analysis to descriptively analyse the process trends. Prediction models using partial least squares, orthogonal PLS, and principal component regression made it possible to predict the culture viability with model accuracies of 90% or higher.

Critical information can also be generated from pH measurements performed offline. A good example is presented where pH probe signals from bioreactors are corrected after the sterilization operation, but also to compensate for signal drift [14]. This novel non-invasive method to determine pH and pCO2 in bioreactors can be carried out without offline measurements by computation of the chemical correlation between carbon dioxide in the gas phase, dissolved carbon dioxide, bicarbonate, and dependent proton concentrations. The method enables accurate determination of the true pH in the bioreactor without sampling.

Convenient offline sampling of critical process data can also be achieved by employing new sensor fabrication technology. An example of this is shown with screen-printed enzyme-based electrochemical sensors for lactate monitoring in bioreactors [15]. These sensors have huge potential to enable low-cost off-line monitoring of, for example, overflow metabolites in bioprocesses. Here, the design of such a single-use electrochemical biosensor is evaluated. Several aspects of its fabrication and use are addressed, such as the importance of enzyme immobilization, stability, shelf-life, and reproducibility of the sensor.

Bioprocess computation of measurement signals requires successful integration and automation of the analytical procedures. Although well established in industry, pivotal improvements are required to address process analytical goals [16]. The shortcomings of automation are much due to the difficulty with the performance of the sampling procedure, sample preparation, and sample transfer to analysers; and very importantly, to correlate all data with the process and the sampling times. This is challenged in a study with an automated sampling system where the performance of data management software was performed with HPLC for measurement of vitamins and amino acids in combination with a biochemical analyser.

In essence, new process analytical technologies are permanently seeing the daylight. The methods highlighted in this special issue add new resources to bioprocess technology in line with the current industrial needs and where analytical principles are refined with new computational capacities and technological advancements.

Institutional Review Board Statement: Not applicable.

Informed Consent Statement: Not applicable.

Data Availability Statement: Not applicable.

Conflicts of Interest: The author declares no conflict of interest.

References

1. Schügerl, K.; Hubbuch, J. Integrated bioprocesses. *Curr. Opion. Microbiol.* **2005**, *8*, 294–300. [CrossRef] [PubMed]
2. Karst, D.J.; Steinebach, F.; Morbidelli, M. Continuous integrated manufacturing of therapeutic proteins. *Curr. Opin. Biotechnol.* **2018**, *53*, 76–84. [CrossRef] [PubMed]
3. Huang, P.Y.; Lin, Y.; Duffy, B.; Varma, A. In integrated bioprocess for antibodies: From harvest to purified bulk in six hours. *Bioproc. Internal.* **2019**. Available online: https://bioprocessintl.com/2019/an-integrated-bioprocess-for-antibodies-from-harvest-to-purified-bulk-in-six-hours/ (accessed on 13 January 2021).
4. Randek, J.; Mandenius, C.F. On-line soft sensing in upstream bioprocessing. *Crit. Rev. Biotechnol.* **2018**, *38*, 106–121. [CrossRef] [PubMed]
5. Roch, P.; Mandenius, C.F. On-line monitoring of downstream bioprocesses. *Curr. Opin. Chem. Eng.* **2016**, *14*, 112–120. [CrossRef]
6. Elfert, T.; Elsen, K.; Maiwald, M.; Herwig, C. Current and future requirements to industrial analytical infrastructure-part 2: Smart sensors. *Anal. Bioanal. Chem.* **2020**, *412*, 2037–2045. [CrossRef] [PubMed]
7. Goldrick, S.; Sandner, V.; Cheeks, M.; Turner, R.; Farid, S.S.; McCreath, G.; Glassey, J. Multivariate data analysis methodology to solve data challenges related to scale-up model validation and missing data on a micro-bioreactor system. *Biotechnol. J.* **2020**, *15*, 1800684. [CrossRef] [PubMed]
8. Glassey, J.; Gernaey, K.V.; Oliveria, R.; Striedner, G.; Clemens, C.; Schultz, T.V.; Mandenius, C.F. Process analytical technology (PAT) for biopharmaceuticals. *Biotechnol. J.* **2011**, *6*, 369–377. [CrossRef] [PubMed]
9. Pais, D.A.M.; Galrao, P.R.S.; Kryzhanska, A.; Barbau, J.; Isidro, I.A.; Alves, P.M. Holographic imaging of insect cell cultures: Online non-invasive monitoring of adeno-associated virus production and cell concentration. *Processes* **2020**, *8*, 487. [CrossRef]

10. Tran, T.; Eskilson, O.; Mayer, F.; Gustavsson, R.; Selegård, R.; Lundström, I.; Mandenius, C.F.; Martinsson, E.; Aili, D. Real-time nanoplasmonic sensor for IgG monitoring in bioproduction. *Processes* **2020**, *8*, 1302. [CrossRef]
11. Goldrick, S.; Umprecht, A.; Tang, A.; Zakrzewski, R.; Cheeks, R.; Turner, R.; Charles, A.; Les, K.; Hulley, M.; Spencer, C.; et al. High-throughput Raman spectroscopy combined with innovate data analysis workflow to enhance biopharmaceutical process development. *Processes* **2020**, *8*, 1179. [CrossRef]
12. Pais, D.A.M.; Brown, C.; Neuman, A.; Mathur, K.; Isidro, I.A.; Alves, P.M.; Slade, P.G. Dielectric spectroscopy to improve the production of 2 rAAV used in Gene Therapy. *Processes* **2020**, *8*, 1456. [CrossRef]
13. Doppler, P.; Veiter, L.; Spaduit, O.; Herwig, C.; Rajamanickam, V. A chemometric tool to monitor and predict cell viability in filamentous fungi bioprocesses using UV chromatogram fingerprints. *Processes* **2020**, *8*, 461. [CrossRef]
14. Klinger, C.; Trinkaus, V.; Wallocha, T. Novel carbon dioxide-based method for accurate determination of pH and pCO$_2$ in mammalian cell culture processes. *Processes* **2020**, *8*, 520. [CrossRef]
15. Theuer, L.; Randek, J.; Junne, S.; Neubauer, P.; Mandenius, C.F.; Beni, V. Single-use printed biosensor for L-lactate and its application in bioprocess monitoring. *Processes* **2020**, *8*, 321. [CrossRef]
16. Hofer, A.; Kroll, P.; Barmettler, M.; Herwig, C. A reliable automated sampling system for online and real-time monitoring of CHO cultures. *Processes* **2020**, *8*, 637. [CrossRef]

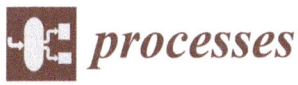

Article

Single-Use Printed Biosensor for L-Lactate and Its Application in Bioprocess Monitoring

Lorenz Theuer [1,†], Judit Randek [2,†], Stefan Junne [3], Peter Neubauer [3], Carl-Fredrik Mandenius [2,*] and Valerio Beni [1]

1. Department of Printed Electronics, RISE Acreo, Research Institute of Sweden, 60221 Norrköping, Sweden; lorenz.theuer@ri.se (L.T.); Valerio.Beni@ri.se (V.B.)
2. Division of Biotechnology, IFM, Linköping University, 58183 Linköping, Sweden; judit.randek@liu.se
3. Department of Bioprocess Engineering, Technische Universität Berlin, 13355 Berlin, Germany; stefan.junne@tu-berlin.de (S.J.); peter.neubauer@tu-berlin.de (P.N.)
* Correspondence: carl-fredrik.mandenius@liu.se
† Shared first authors.

Received: 12 February 2020; Accepted: 4 March 2020; Published: 9 March 2020

Abstract: There is a profound need in bioprocess manufacturing for low-cost single-use sensors that allow timely monitoring of critical product and production attributes. One such opportunity is screen-printed enzyme-based electrochemical sensors, which have the potential to enable low-cost online and/or off-line monitoring of specific parameters in bioprocesses. In this study, such a single-use electrochemical biosensor for lactate monitoring is designed and evaluated. Several aspects of its fabrication and use are addressed, including enzyme immobilization, stability, shelf-life and reproducibility. Applicability of the biosensor to off-line monitoring of bioprocesses was shown by testing in two common industrial bioprocesses in which lactate is a critical quality attribute (*Corynebacterium* fermentation and mammalian Chinese hamster ovary (CHO) cell cultivation). The specific response to lactate of the screen-printed biosensor was characterized by amperometric measurements. The usability of the sensor at typical industrial culture conditions was favorably evaluated and benchmarked with commonly used standard methods (HPLC and enzymatic kits). The single-use biosensor allowed fast and accurate detection of lactate in prediluted culture media used in industrial practice. The design and fabrication of the biosensor could most likely be adapted to several other critical bioprocess analytes using other specific enzymes. This makes this single-use screen-printed biosensor concept a potentially interesting and versatile tool for further applications in bioprocess monitoring.

Keywords: lactate biosensor; enzyme electrode; off-line monitoring; screen-printing; at-line measurement; in-line monitoring

1. Introduction

The need for sensors that can contribute to make biological production more efficient and better controlled is profound [1–3]. Sensors able to monitor critical process events in close to real time are especially needed. This includes changes in concentrations of critical process parameters (CPPs) and critical quality attributes (CQAs) that enable active control to ensure optimal production conditions of the bioprocess [2]. Examples are (i) metabolites that control metabolic flow rates of the target end-product or (ii) overflow metabolites of the central pathways, such as acetate, ethanol and lactate [4]. If these analytes can be monitored in time, cellular growth and expression of target products can be enhanced [5].

As industrial microbial and cell cultures are slow growing processes, it is sufficient to measure these analytes intermittently at the process line and to take appropriate control actions based on the measurement results [6]. However, the procedures require sensors that are easy to handle, cost-effective and accurate enough for the purpose of the corrective control action. Examples of efforts in applying such sensors for monitoring of bioprocesses and cell cultures have recently been reported [7–9].

Currently, commercial alternatives are available, such as high-pressure liquid chromatography (HPLC), enzyme kits and sensors for medical care [10], some with excellent sensitivity, which is important in many medical applications, but less essential in bioprocesses. Although, these alternatives require either high investments or extensive maintenance or time-consuming analytical procedures; still, their analytical performances may be insufficient.

Biosensors, with their inherent enzymatic specificity towards certain metabolites and their favorable analytical performance in biological fluids, have slowly gained acceptance in a variety of fields including clinical, food and environmental analysis [10–12]. Among the signal transduction methods applied with biosensors, the electrochemical biosensors are highly attractive due to their suitability for miniaturization, mass production and low-cost manufacturability (e.g., by printing techniques) [13,14].

The interest in low-cost sensors has significantly boosted the interest in printing; for example, roll-to-roll and gravure printing have been increasingly reported for the manufacturing of electrochemical biosensors [15]. Together with an enhanced importance of the single-use approach, these techniques present regulatory advantages, including transparent conditions for implementation, distribution, storage and reproducible validation [16].

A plethora of electrochemical lactate biosensor designs has previously been presented for applications in medicine and biotechnology [17–20]. The majority of these rely on the use of enzymes such as lactate oxidase or lactate dehydrogenase incorporated in a supporting membrane [21].

Despite clinical analysis having been the most explored application for lactate biosensors, reports on this technology for cell culture monitoring have also been presented. For example, Boero and colleagues [7] reported on fabrication via thin film technology of a dual sensing system for on-line monitoring of glucose and lactate in pharmaceutical processes. The same authors reported on a screen-printed electrochemical biosensor based on carbon-nanotube-modified carbon electrodes for the detection of glucose and lactate in an SN56 cell culture [22]. Later, Li and colleagues [8] reported on continuous monitoring of extracellular lactate in cardiac cell culture using an electrochemical biosensor based on lactate dehydrogenase with methylene green on nanotubes.

The requirements on lactate measurements vary considerably in medical applications, drug manufacturing and bioproduction regarding validation, clinical safety and reliability. For industrial bioprocess applications, as addressed here, lactate measurement at higher levels (e.g., 5–35 µM) are of decisive value for the process performance [23]. Furthermore, compliance of these sensors with good manufacturing practice (GMP) guidelines, validation criteria and specific needs at the production plant are important requirements which also must be met.

In this article we present a novel design for a single-use screen-printed lactate biosensor based on a fabrication method easy to mass produce. The sensor is intended for use at-line in bioprocesses, such as mammalian cell cultivations for biopharmaceuticals and bacterial cultivations for primary metabolites and heterologous protein production. The specific enzyme used in the sensor, lactate oxidase, was immobilized onto a polyethylene terephthalate foil, creating a recognition element of high specificity, acceptable stability and low enzyme cost. This lactate biosensor design exhibited promising and reliable data, both in bacterial and mammalian cell cultures, when used in typical cell cultivation media.

2. Materials and Methods

2.1. Single-Use Biosensor Fabrication

2.1.1. Printing

The electrochemical strips, in the two-electrode configuration, used for the assembly of the single-use biosensor were fabricated by screen-printing onto a 125 µm thick polyethylene terephthalate (PET) substrate foil (Polyfoil Bias). To minimize deformation of the substrate foil during the printing process, the PET substrate underwent a thermal pretreatment (140 °C for 45 min). The printing procedure consisted of four consecutive steps: (1) printing of the conductive tracks using a commercial silver ink (Ag5000, DuPont, UK), followed by its thermal curing (180 s at 130 °C); (2) printing and thermal curing (180 s at 130 °C) of the Ag/AgCl reference/counter electrode (C61003P7, Gwent, UK); (3) printing and curing (180 s at 120 °C) of the carbon working electrode (7102, DuPont, UK); (4) coating the sensor electrodes with two layers of a UV-curable dielectric layer (5018, DuPont, UK) in order to ensure that only the sensing area (working electrode and reference/counter electrode) and the connecting pads at the far end of the Ag conductive tracks were exposed (see Figure 1b). A semiautomatic screen printer (DEK Horizon 03i printer, ASM Assembly Systems GmbH, Germany) was used to fabricate the strips. The final electrochemical strips had a working electrode with an area of 0.0177 cm^2 (geometrical) and a counter/reference electrode with an area of 0.212 cm^2 (about 12 times that of the working electrode area). Each sheet (A4 area) contained 108 strips.

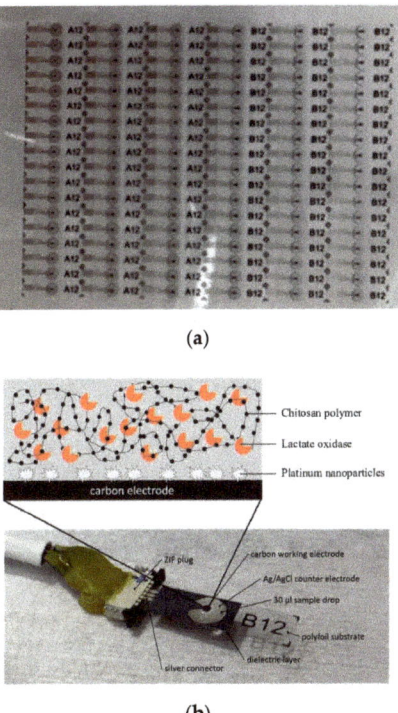

Figure 1. (a) An A4-sheet containing 108 screen-printed electrochemical sensors for biosensor development; (b) the fabricated electrochemical biosensor. The insert shows the architecture of the enzyme layer with the Pt-nanoparticle-modified carbon electrode surface covered by the enzyme/chitosan membrane.

2.1.2. Biosensor Assembling

Prior to the immobilization of the enzyme, the working electrode, where sensing takes place, underwent an activation step and a metallization step. Activation of the electrode was carried out by potential cycling (0 to 1.5 V, scan rate 50 mV s^{-1}) applied to it 25 times, with the strips immersed in a 10 mM PBS buffer. The working electrode was subsequently modified by platinum nanoparticles (Pt-NPs) that performed catalytic oxidation of H_2O_2 formed at enzymatic oxidation of lactate. The Pt-NPs were electrodeposited onto the working electrode following a two-step process inspired by the protocol previously reported by Diacci et al. [24] where Pt-NPs were deposited by applying one drop (ca. 30 µL) of a 1 mM solution of K_2PtCl_6 in 0.1 M KCl and by sequential pulsing a potential of 0.5 V for 0.01 s followed by −0.7 V for 10 s for 25 cycles.

Subsequently, the sensors with the deposited Pt-NPs were coated with the enzyme-containing membrane. Chitosan membrane was prepared adapting previously reported protocols [25,26]. The membrane was prepared by dissolving 0.1 wt% of chitosan in 0.1 M HCl at 80–90 °C for 2 h. The pH of the obtained chitosan solution was adjusted to 4.5 before the solution was filtered through a 0.45 µm syringe filter and stored at 4 °C.

Dry lactate oxidase (Sigma Aldrich) was subsequently dissolved in PBS at a concentration of 200 U/mL. Different dilutions of the enzyme stock solution were prepared and mixed with the chitosan solution in 3:4 (enzyme:chitosan) proportion to obtain the desired enzyme concentration on the sensor surface. A drop of 2 µL of the mixture was cast onto the working electrode and left to dry for 2 h at room temperature. These enzyme sensor strips were stored at 4 °C until use.

2.1.3. Characterization of the Single-Use Biosensor

Cyclic voltammetry was used to characterize the sensors. Sensor strips were recorded (−0.4 to 0.6 V at a scan rate 50 mV s^{-1}) before and after modification of the Pt nanoparticles to evaluate the electroactivity of different culture media.

Chronoamperometric measurements (0.4 V for 180 s) were used for lactate detection in both laboratory solutions and culture samples. The current was recorded after 180 s in all of the chronoamperometric measurements.

Electrochemical measurements of culture samples were performed by dropping 35 µL of the sample onto the electrode.

When the sensors were recorded for 24-h periods, the sensors were immersed in a beaker with PBS containing L-lactate at different concentrations. This procedure was used to (i) minimize the effect of evaporation and (ii) reduce influence of substrate depletion and/or product accumulation.

Prior to measurement of lactate in culture samples a precalibration of the sensor was carried out either in culture media or diluted PBS.

2.2. Cell Cultivation Processes

2.2.1. Corynebacterium Cultivation

A *Corynebacterium* strain DM1945 $\Delta act3$:P_{tuf}-$ldcC_{OPT}$ [27,28] was precultivated in two consecutive steps (I and II) before running the batch culture in which the sensors were evaluated.

Preculture I was carried out in an LB medium (50 mL supplemented with 22 g/L glucose) with 200 µL of the cryo-preserved *C. glutamicum* added. After 4 h at 30 °C of cultivation, using an orbital shaker with an amplitude of 70 mm at 200 rpm, the cells were transferred to Preculture II.

Preculture II was carried out in CgXII medium (85 mL supplemented with 24 g/L glucose) seeded with 15 mL of Preculture I using a procedure described by Keilhauer et al. [29]. Preculture II was cultured for 20 h at 30 °C in a rotary incubator at 200 rpm.

Subsequently, 10 mL of Preculture II was transferred to a shake-flask (batch) with the same CgXII medium (50 mL supplemented with 24 g/L glucose). The batch culture was run for 7 h at 30 °C in a rotary incubator using intermittent shaking with 15 min off/on intervals.

Samples were collected once per hour and centrifuged; the supernatant was frozen at −20 °C prior to lactate analysis. Dry cell mass was determined by duplicates gravimetrically.

2.2.2. Chinese Hamster Ovary (CHO) Cell Cultivation with RPMI Medium

CHO cells (CHO-K1 (ACC 110, DSMZ)) were cultured for seven days in 500 mL shake-flasks (batch) containing 100 mL of RPMI medium with an initial glucose concentration of 20 g/L glucose. The cultivations were run in a CO_2-incubator on a shaker at 50 rpm, at 37 °C and 5% CO_2.

Samples were taken once per day, centrifuged, sterile filtered and stored in a freezer at −20 °C until measurement. The collected samples were thawed and analyzed using the single-use biosensor and, in parallel, measured by HPLC for correlation of the single-use biosensor readings.

Cell counts were carried out by microscopy using a Neubauer chamber. Between 300 and 1000 cells were counted in each sample. To assess cell viability, trypan-blue staining was applied.

2.2.3. Chinese Ovary Hamster (CHO) Cell Cultivation with Proprietary Medium

Another Chinese hamster ovary (CHO) cell line was provided by Fujifilm Diosynth Biotechnologies (Billingham, UK). The cells were cultured in 500 mL spinner-flasks for 13 days by intermittent addition of fresh culture medium supplemented with glutamine and antibiotic specially designed for the CHO cell line (proprietary medium provided by Fujifilm Diosynth Biotechnologies). Cultivations were run in a CO_2-incubator at 5% CO_2 and 36.5 °C and using a stirrer speed of 50 rpm. The initial starting concentration of the cells was 200,000 cells/mL in a volume of 350 mL.

Samples were taken once per day and centrifuged; the supernatant was stored at −20 °C until measurement. The collected samples were thawed and analyzed using the single-use biosensor and, in parallel, measured by a Megazyme lactate kit for determining the correlation of the single-use biosensor readings. Cell number was determined by staining with trypan-blue and manually counting in a light microscope using a Bürker chamber.

2.3. Measurement of Lactate with the Single-Use Biosensor

In order to evaluate the applicability of the single-use printed biosensor, the following measurement/correlation protocol was used.

The L-lactate content in the diluted sample was measured by using three different biosensors. Concentration of the L-lactate in the sample was then calculated by fitting the obtained sensor's reading in a calibration curve, which was made from five single-use biosensors (calibration points: 50, 275 and 500 µM). The samples (35 µL) were pipetted on the measurement area of the sensor.

The proposed biosensor is based on the FAD-mediated enzymatic oxidation of L-lactate (1 and 2) followed by electrocatalytic detection of hydrogen peroxide (3) formed in stoichiometry proportions to lactate. The sensitive and stable detection of H_2O_2 at the sensor surface is crucial for proper function of the sensor.

$$\text{L-lactate} + FAD_{(LOx)} \rightarrow \text{Pyruvate} + FADH_{2(LOx)} \tag{1}$$

$$FADH_{2(LOx)} + O_2 \rightarrow H_2O_2 + FAD_{(LOx)} \tag{2}$$

$$H_2O_2 \rightarrow 2H^+ + O_2 + 2e^- \tag{3}$$

2.4. Measurement of Lactate with Reference Methods

2.4.1. High-Performance Liquid Chromatography

Samples were filtered through a membrane filter with a pore size of 0.8 µm (Carl Roth, Karlsruhe, Germany) directly after sampling. The supernatant was transferred to 1.5 mL tubes, immediately stored at −80 °C and thawed before measurements.

The concentration of L-lactate in culture's samples (supernatant) was obtained by HPLC with an Agilent 1200 system (Waldbronn, Germany) equipped with a refractive index detector and a

HyperRezTM XP Carbohydrate H+ column (300 × 7.7 mm, 8 µm) (Fisher Scientific, Schwerte, Germany) using 0.1 M H_2SO_4 as carrier solution at a flow rate of 0.5 mL min^{-1} and a temperature of 15 °C [28,30]. The HPLC method had an LOD of 1 µM. Measurement data were analyzed with the Agilent Chemstation for LC 3D systems software Rev. B.04.01.

2.4.2. Ultraviolet Spectroscopy

Samples were thawed and diluted 1:60 with PBS. The L-lactate concentration was obtained using a lactate kit (Megazyme, Ireland) according to product instructions. The assay had a linear range between 34 and 225 µM and an LOD of 2.36 µM. UV spectra (340 nm) were recorded with an Ultraspec 1000 UV/VIS spectrophotometer (Pharmacia Biotech, UK).

3. Results and Discussion

The optimization of the fabrication procedure of the single-use lactate biosensor, the evaluation of its storage and operation stabilities and its analytical performances in a variety of relevant crude media are detailed below. Finally, data are presented from two types of cultivations that are commonly applied in industry.

3.1. Sensor Fabrication and Functionalization

In order to evaluate the feasibility of the screen-printing method for the manufacturing of the electrochemical sensor suitable as a platform for enzyme immobilization, and for demonstrating the possibility of its mass-production, ten sheets with 108 sensor strips on each were fabricated (Figure 1a). The fabrication yield (defined as the percent of sensors with individually addressable electrodes) was estimated by optical inspection and electrical verification to be 92%. This number was not considered an optimal value of the method per se but was an indicator that the sensors had the necessary prerequisites for being developed into a reliable single-use enzyme sensor.

For the purpose of the study, it was an important indication that the manufacturing process had enough robustness for further development.

In order to enable this catalytic oxidation with high efficiency, the carbon surface of the sensor electrode was functionalized by platinum nanoparticles (Pt-NPs) using the procedure described in Section 2.1.2.

Importantly, as can be seen in Figure 2a, no electrochemical response was recorded at the bare carbon electrode (black line); while when Pt-NPs (blue-colored line) (without enzyme) were electrodeposited onto the electrode surface, distinct and significant redox reactions related to the oxidation and reduction of H_2O_2 were recorded. Based on the transient shape of the CV-curve, an applied potential of 0.4 V (vs. internal Ag/AgCl reference electrode) was chosen for the subsequent amperometric measurements.

As demonstrated above, the electrocatalytic ability of the Pt-NP-modified carbon electrode to detect H_2O_2 makes it feasible to assemble the biosensor by further modifying its composite Pt-NP surface with an Lox-containing chitosan membrane. As a first step, the biosensor surface was provided with increasing loading of LOx (5, 10, 20 and 40 U) in the membrane. These membranes were prepared to identify a favorable and optimal LOx concentration.

The optimal concentration was considered to be the one that would allow to widen the linear range of the sensor (towards high concentration) and to provide an easily recordable electrochemical response. As expected, the increase of LOx loading in the membrane resulted in an increase of the biosensor response (Appendix A Figure A1). However, this did not result in any significant improvement in the linear dynamic range of the sensor. Subsequently, in a compromise between the sensor response and its costs, an LOx loading of 20 U in the membrane was selected for the measurements.

Based on the electrocatalytic effect of the Pt-NPs, which was observed as described above by cyclic voltammetry (Figure 2a), and the selected enzyme composition of the membrane, a set of biosensors (ca. 20 units) were fabricated and their reproducibility and stability during storage and at operation were both evaluated. As can be seen in Figure 2b, good reproducibility of these biosensors was achieved, as proven by the low standard deviation obtained at calibration in pure laboratory solutions (PBS) (at 0 to 500 µM L-lactate using 10 sensors).

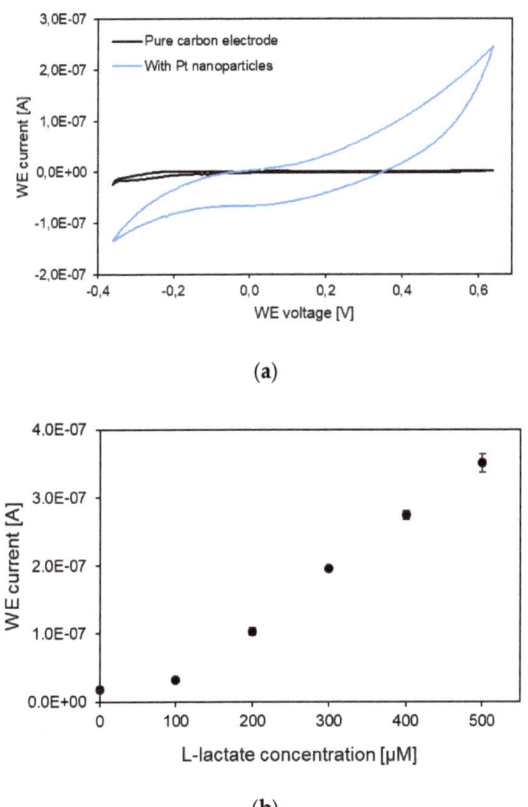

Figure 2. (a) Cyclic voltammetry in 50 µM H_2O_2, dissolved in PBS at a 25 mV/s scanning rate with a bare carbon electrode and a carbon electrode with electrodeposited Pt-NPs; (b) calibration curve of a L-lactate biosensor in PBS. The standard deviation was calculated using the response of ten biosensors.

The operational and storage stability of the biosensors were evaluated with the purpose of gaining better understanding of their applicability for off-line or at-line bioreactor monitoring. As seen in Figure 3a, the electrochemical response of the biosensor was rapidly degrading when applied in continuous measurement mode with a fast decrease, especially after the first hour, which was followed by a continuous drift of the signal amplitude. This result clearly highlights the inappropriateness of using the developed biosensors for continuous real-time monitoring in bioreactors. However, the observed stability is still adequate for the application of the sensor in off-line single-use modality.

From Figure 2b, it is evident that the high level of reproducibility of freshly prepared sensors allows their off-line single-use utilization. A further aspect to be evaluated to ensure the biosensor applicability during cultivation (for two weeks) is its stability upon storage. To test this, a batch of biosensors (44 units) were fabricated the same day, using the same stock solution of enzyme membrane, and stored either dry at room temperature (21 °C) or at 4 °C in closed petri dishes. Prior to testing, biosensors where transferred to room temperature and washed with PBS (to hydrate the membrane). Then, these sensors were used for measuring amperometrically a 500 µM solution of L-lactate in PBS.

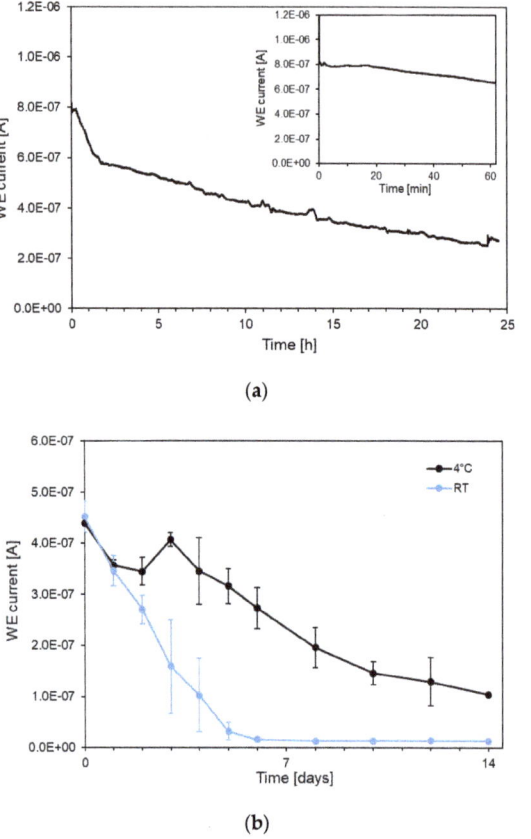

Figure 3. (a) Continuous reading of the biosensor for 24 h (the first hour inserted) in 500 µM L-lactate PBS solution; (b) stability of the biosensors upon storage (14 days) in dry conditions at 4 °C and at room temperature (21 °C). All readings were performed in PBS solutions containing 500 µM of L-lactate.

As seen in Figure 3b, sensor units stored at room temperature quickly lost their response, and no activity could be recorded after 6 days. Similarly, the sensor units stored at 4 °C lost their activity upon storage, even if the loss was partial (after 14 days, about 30% of the performance at day 1 was recorded). No significant improvements in stability resulted from other storage conditions: (i) in dry state at −20 °C; (ii) in liquid state in PBS at 4 °C; (iii) in PBS containing 250 µM lactate at 4 °C (Appendix A Figure A2). Thus, stability of the sensor is short, suggesting that the immobilization technique should be further refined. Previous experiences of enzyme immobilization in hydrogels may inform such procedures [31].

3.2. Characterization of the Electrochemical Behaviour of Culture Media

Prior to applying the developed single-use biosensors to monitor bacterial and cell cultures, electrochemical characterization of the biosensors in typical culture media was performed; this evaluation was needed to identify potential interferences from media components in the electrochemical surface process (e.g., redox processes overlapping those of H_2O_2).

Electrochemical responses in the culture media to be used in the subsequent off-line testing of the sensors were systematically recorded in presence or absence of H_2O_2 and using bare carbon electrodes or Pt-NP-covered electrodes. The media investigated were as follows: (i) an industrial culture medium (proprietary medium from Fujifilm Diosynth Biotechnologies; in dilution 1:60 with PBS); (ii) RPMI media; (iii) a CGXII medium.

As seen in Figure 4, no significant electrochemical interferences were recorded for the industrial cell culture medium (Figure 4a) and the RPMI medium (Figure 4b); on the other end, in these media the catalytic oxidation of the H_2O_2 seems to be significantly inhibited.

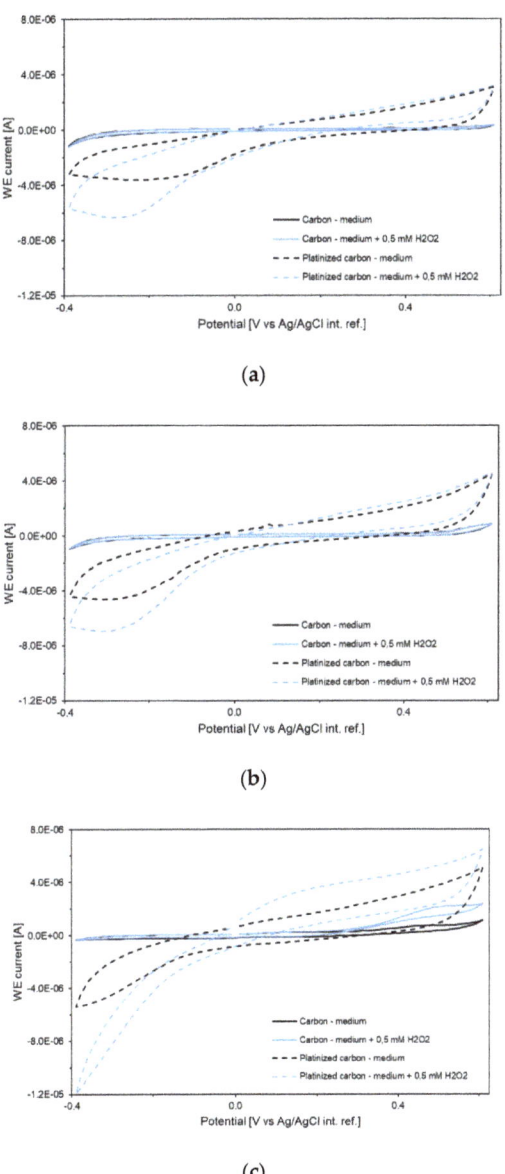

Figure 4. Cyclic voltammetry measurements in three cell culture media using bare and Pt-NP-functionalized carbon electrodes in the absence or presence of 500 µM H_2O_2. (**a**) Fujifilm media diluted 1 to 60 in PBS; (**b**) RPMI medium; (**c**) CGXII medium. Voltage is cycled between −0.4 and 0.6 V at a rate of 50 mV/s with a voltage step of 10 mV.

In the case of the CGXII medium (Figure 4c), an intrinsic electrochemical activity was recorded at the bare carbon electrode (full black line); however, this response was significantly smaller than those recorded for H_2O_2 at both bare carbon electrode (full blue line) and Pt-NP-covered electrode (dotted blue line). The results shown in Figure 4 confirm that electrochemical measurements are feasible in the investigated media.

It should be noted however, that the measurement of L-lactate in the culture medium was significantly affected by poor reproducibility, as seen in data in Appendix A Figure A3, in which the calibration curves carried out in RPMI medium and PBS are also shown for comparison. The analytical performance of the biosensor in the investigated media is summarized in Table 1.

Table 1. Analytical performance of the developed biosensor in the different media.

	PBS Diluted Fujifilm Media	RPMI	DGXII
Sensitivity (A/µM)	7.64×10^{-10}	6.27×10^{-10}	5.3×10^{-10}
LOD (µM)	10	67	101

3.3. Application of the Printed Single-Use Biosensor in Microbial and Mammlian Cell Cultivation Monitoring

Based on the findings in Sections 3.1 and 3.2, it is concluded that application of printed single-use biosensors in cell culture analysis is possible, but only by applying an off-line single-use approach. It was also obvious from the results that careful precalibration is needed in order to compensate for storage-related losses and for effects of the media composition. Furthermore, the limited linear range of the biosensors requires dilution of cultivation samples to bring the concentrations of L-lactate within the detectable sensitivity window of the biosensor. This need for dilution of cell culture samples prior to measurement has been previously been discussed by other authors [22].

3.3.1. *Corynebacterium glutamicum* Cultivation

Prior to lactate analysis of samples from *C. glutamicum* cultures, five freshly fabricated biosensor units were used carry out a three-point calibration in the range 0 to 500 µM of L-lactate in CGXII media. Each biosensor was used three times from lower to higher concentrations. The L-lactate concentrations in the sample were calculated by fitting the off-line biosensor response to this calibration.

In order to reach the dynamic L-lactate concentration range of the biosensor, the samples were diluted 1 to 42 (decided according to data available from previous cultivations) in CGXII media. Eight biosensors were used (each of them three times) in alternating order to determine the lactate concentration of the samples. The first readings of each biosensor have been recorded separately (1× sensor) to be able to study the effect of multiple use on accuracy.

As seen in Figure 5, the values calculated using the single-use biosensor measurements coincided well with those recorded by HPLC.

At low L-lactate concentrations (<5 mM), the measurements of the single-use biosensors underestimate the concentrations; at higher concentrations (>5 mM) the measurements have high standard deviation.

The negative L-lactate concentrations can be explained by the fact that the measurements, as a result of the dilution, are very close to the limit of detection (0.101 mM) of the biosensor in the CGXII media. This is not a significant problem from a process-monitoring perspective, since the relevant information is in the higher concentrations of L-lactate in the cell culture.

The high standard deviation is a result of two interconnected effects: (1) being close to the limit of linearity (above 0.6 mM) and (2) the calibration method. These, together with the multiple usage of the biosensor, lead to saturation of the enzymes on the sensor surface, increasing the signal after each measurement and making multiple readings impossible. This explanation is also supported by the graph of the single-fold (1x) biosensor measurements (Figure 5), where the fresh biosensors show slightly higher concentrations than HPLC, while the threefold-measured mean biosensor values show slightly less response.

In order to achieve a better monitoring performance and accuracy, different calibration methods were compared in the upcoming cultivations.

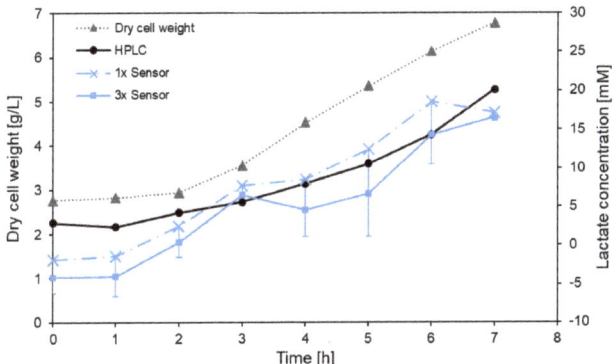

Figure 5. Monitoring of lactate off-line for seven hours of *C. glutamicum* cultivation in CGXII medium using the single-use biosensor, and its comparison with off-line HPLC lactate measurements. The 1× graph shows the first recordings with individual biosensors. The 3× graph shows the mean value of recordings of three individual thrice-used biosensors. The cultivation chart also shows the growth of the bacteria as dry cell weight concentrations.

3.3.2. Mammalian Cell (CHO) Culture

In order to demonstrate the versatility of the single-use biosensor, CHO cells were cultured according to two different procedures: in one procedure the cells were cultured for seven days in shake-flasks as batch cultures using RPMI medium (see procedure described in Section 2.2.2); in another procedure the cells were cultured for 13 days in larger spinner-flasks as fed-batch cultures using an industrial culture medium (see procedure in Section 2.2.3). The collected frozen samples were thawed and analyzed by the single-use biosensor and, in parallel, either analyzed by HPLC (first procedure) or by a colorimetric lactate enzyme assay (second procedure) for correlation of the biosensor readings.

Prior to analysis, all samples were diluted 1 to 55 (dilution factor defined according to pre-existing data) in the RPMI medium, or 1 to 60 in PBS for the industrial medium (as shown feasible in preliminary tests), to reach the dynamic range for lactate of the single-use biosensor. With the aim to improve the accuracy of the biosensor measurement, two other calibration methods, a two-point calibration and a cross-calibration, were compared with linear calibration when used in RPMI medium.

In the cross-calibration approach, each biosensor was used to measure the start sample, the end point sample and a third sample in between these two samples. The results of the HPLC measurements (start and end points) were used to cross-calibrate each biosensor separately. L-lactate values of the third sample were calculated based on a linear regression of the two-point cross-calibration. As seen in Figure 6a, linear calibration, either with the single or multiple use of the biosensors, shows lower responses than HPLC in the previous bacterial cultivations.

The two-point calibration using two biosensors proved inaccurate, while cross-calibration using the HPLC measurements showed better accuracy, both at lower and higher concentrations. Thus, the cross-calibration method was used to calibrate the single-use biosensors in the first CHO procedure.

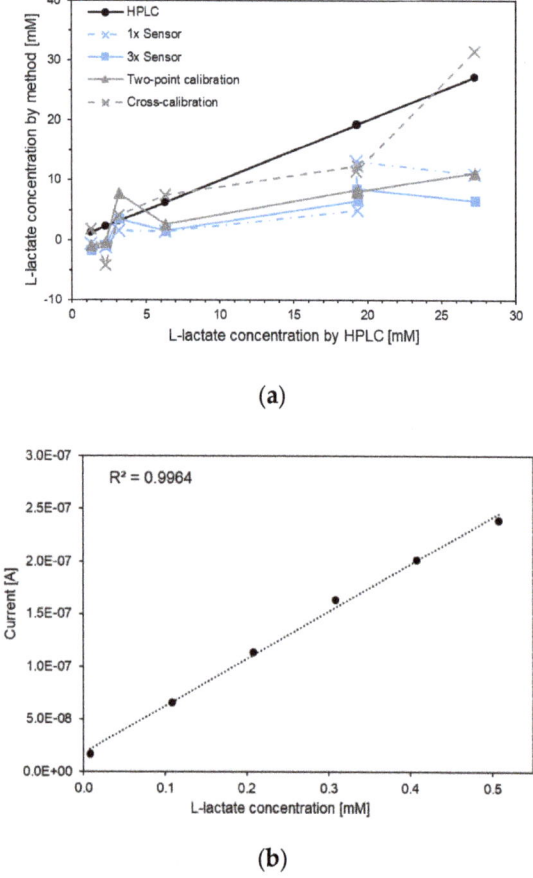

Figure 6. (a) The correlation of the different calibration methods with the HPLC measurements. The lactate measurements of the HPLC have been compared with the measurements of single and multiple use of the biosensors, two-point calibration and cross-calibration. (b) Five-point calibration in the industrial medium.

With lactate samples collected from the CHO culture performed in the industrial medium, a five-point calibration was carried out (Figure 6b). The biosensor response showed good linearity between 0.008 and 0.5 mM. Thus, this calibration method was used in the spinner-flask fed-batch CHO cell cultivation.

In Figure 7a, the correlation between the biosensor and HPLC measurements in the shake-flask batch CHO cell culture is shown. Each datapoint was measured by a separate sensor in a single-use way, as it would be in industrial use. As seen, the correlation is high during this CHO cell cultivation, except in the early phase, where the cell concentration and viability is low and where L-lactate concentrations are close to the limit of detection of the biosensor after sample dilution. Clearly, the biosensors showed an improved accuracy with the cross-calibration method, being able to follow the increasing lactate concentration in a wide range (0–25 mM) shown in the fed-batch culture. This variation of L-lactate concentration also mirrors the expected lactate profile during growth and metabolic overflow in a batch CHO cell culture.

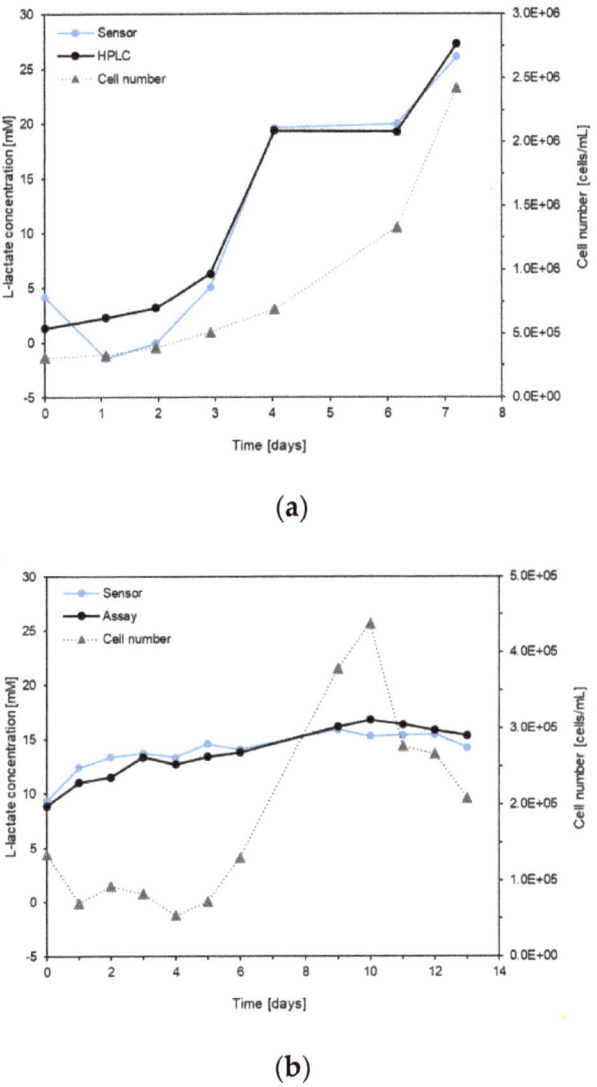

Figure 7. Mammalian cell culture measurements at line using the single-use biosensor. (**a**) Seven-day batch cultivation showing lactate measurements with the single-use biosensor in comparison with off-line HPLC data; (**b**) Thirteen-day fed-batch cultivation showing lactate measurements with the single-use biosensor in comparison with off-line spectroscopic lactate assay data. The growth profiles of CHO cell cultures are shown in (**a**) and (**b**) from viability assays.

In the fed-batch CHO cell cultivation (Figure 7b), higher dilution of the samples than for those from the RPMI medium was necessary, because L-lactate was included as a growth component in the industrial medium.

As seen in Figure 7b, good correlation was also obtained between data from the single-use biosensor and the standard lactate assay. Similarly to the batch CHO cultivation, each datapoint was obtained by a separate sensor. The addition of a higher amount of feed solution to the culture resulted in a drop in cell concentration at the end of the cultivation (day 11 and forward), which is due to the dilution of the culture and not due to cell death (Figure 7b).

The lactate component in the cultivation media is, as expected, produced in a higher amount when the culture is growing (between days 0 and 10), and it stagnates when the cell proliferation retarded (day 11 and onwards). As can be seen in Figure 7b, the biosensor was able to accurately monitor this event in the cultivation.

Evidently, the single-use screen-printed biosensor calibrated with the appropriate method (either five-point or cross-calibration) is able to detect L-lactate in a wide concentration range in various culture media. Its measurement range also covers the typical lactate concentration range (5–35 mM) expected during mammalian processes [23]. Thus, the sensor seems to be a realistic alternative for at-line bioreactor monitoring, providing a convenient and user-friendly low-cost alternative to other sensor methods applied today [32,33].

4. Conclusions

The screen-printed single-use biosensor for lactate bioprocess monitoring developed and evaluated here is convenient to mass-produce at a low batch production cost. The fabrication procedure results in a device unit that shows the necessary sensitivity, reproducibility and, partly, the stability needed for the monitoring of certain bioprocess applications. The developed enzyme sensor with the right calibration method proved to be suitable for the fast screening of different cultivation processes.

Certain needs for improvement can also be mentioned, such as (1) a more extended long-term stability and higher reproducibility of the sensor; (2) access to automated dispensing tools for deposition of the enzyme membrane; and (3) aluminum pouches for sensor storage in controlled atmosphere. These improvements would significantly enhance the performance and shelf-life of the sensor as well as contribute to satisfying regulatory demands. Even without these improvements, however, the sensor can be suitable for internal in-process use as a complement to analytical methods and devices in use today.

The devised fabrication method is expandable to other enzymes. The number of potential applications for biotechnology is vast, e.g., other metabolites prevalent the culture media such as amino acids, other organic acids and alcohols, some main products, other side-products.

The impact of at-line monitoring using single-use biosensors on production efficiency and economy is potentially profound. Total production time and product titer can be optimized under conditions of the chosen process. The printing-based fabrication of the biosensor has the flexibility of a variety/assortment of enzyme variants. Thus, these initial findings may have significant impact and motivate further development.

Author Contributions: L.T. performed development of the fabrication of the printed biosensor. J.R. and L.T. conceived and performed the bioprocess application study. B.V., D.S., M.G. and L.T. conceived the design of the printed device. J.R., L.T., S.J., P.N. and C.-F.M. conceived the study of the application in the two bioprocesses. L.T. and J.R. evaluated the results. J.R., L.T., V.B. and C.-F.M. drafted the manuscript and all co-authors reviewed the manuscript. All authors have read and agreed to the published version of the manuscript.

Funding: This project has received funding from the European Union's Horizon 2020 research and innovation program under the Marie Skłodowska-Curie actions grant agreement No. 643056 (BIORAPID).

Acknowledgments: The authors also thank Fujifilm Diosynth Biotechnologies for providing the CHO cell line and the culture media formulation.

Conflicts of Interest: The authors declare no conflict of interest.

Appendix A

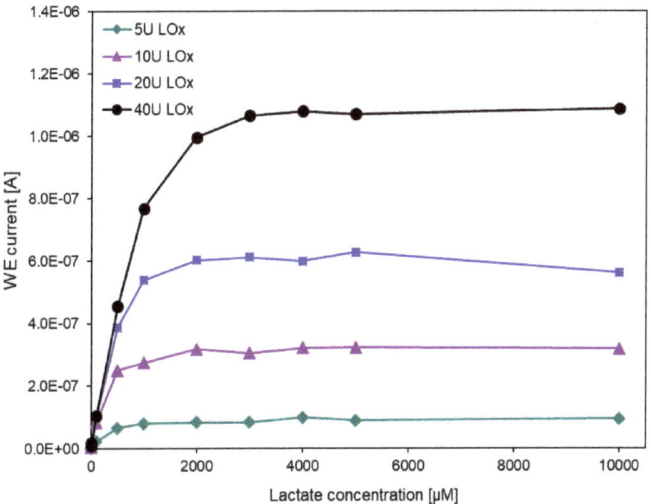

Figure A1. Amperometric L-lactate biosensor calibration curves (at potential 0.4 V and 180 s) in PBS with different enzyme loads on the sensor.

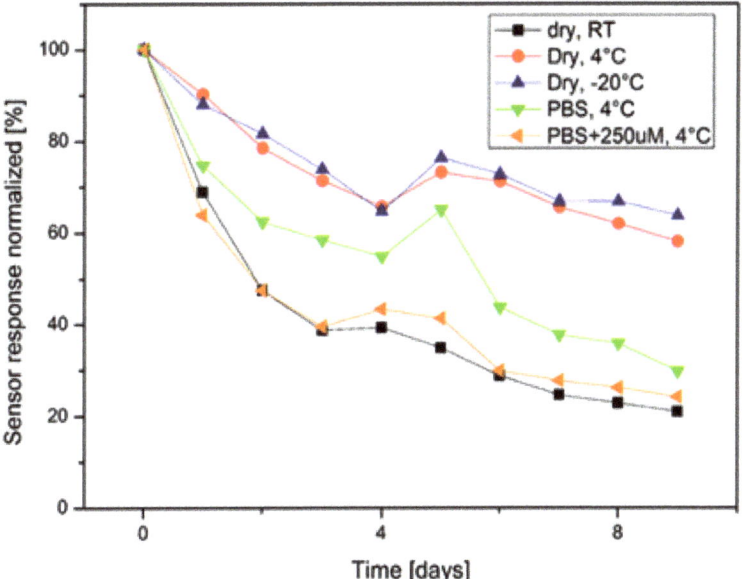

Figure A2. Preliminary comparison of different storing conditions for the biosensor. Response obtained daily in a 500 µM solution of L-lactate in PBS and normalized against response obtained on day 0.

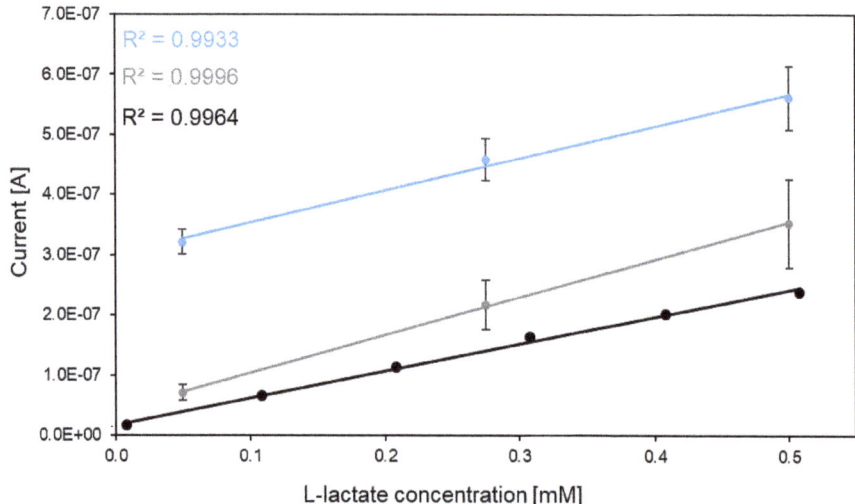

Figure A3. Example of biosensor calibration curve in CGXII medium diluted in PBS (blue line, $n = 5$), RPMI media (grey line, $n = 5$) and Fujifilm media (black line, $n = 1$).

References

1. Alford, J.S. Bioprocess control: Advances and challenges. *Comput. Chem. Eng.* **2006**, *30*, 1464–1475. [CrossRef]
2. Guerra, A.; von Stosch, M.; Glassey, J. Toward biotherapeutic product real-time quality monitoring. *Crit. Rev. Biotechnol.* **2019**, *39*, 289–305. [CrossRef] [PubMed]
3. Randek, J.; Mandenius, C.-F. On-line soft sensing in upstream bioprocessing. *Crit. Rev. Biotechnol.* **2018**, *38*, 106–121. [CrossRef] [PubMed]
4. Schügerl, K. Progress in monitoring, modeling and control of bioprocesses during the last 20 years. *J. Biotechnol.* **2001**, *85*, 149–173. [CrossRef]
5. Villadsen, J.; Nielsen, J.; Lidén, G. Chemicals from metabolic pathways. In *Bioreaction Engineering Principles*; Springer: Berlin, Germany, 2011; pp. 7–62.
6. Sonnleitner, B. Automated measurement and monitoring of bioprocesses: Key elements of the M3C strategy. *Adv. Biochem. Eng. Biotechnol.* **2013**, *132*, 1–33.
7. Boero, C.; Casulli, M.A.; Olivo, J.; Foglia, L.; Orso, E.; Mazza, M.; Carrara, S.; de Micheli, G. Design, development, and validation of an in-situ biosensor array for metabolite monitoring of cell cultures. *Biosens. Bioelectron.* **2014**, *61*, 251–259. [CrossRef]
8. Li, X.; Zhao, L.; Chen, Z.; Lin, Y.; Yu, P.; Mao, L. Continuous electrochemical monitoring of extracellular lactate production from neonatal rat cardiomyocytes following myocardial hypoxia. *Anal. Chem.* **2012**, *84*, 5285–5291. [CrossRef]
9. Mi, S.; Xia, J.; Xu, Y.; Du, Z.; Sun, W. An integrated microchannel biosensor platform to analyse low density lactate metabolism in HepG2 cells in vitro. *RSC Adv.* **2019**, *9*, 9006–9013. [CrossRef]
10. Bahadir, E.B.; Sezginturk, M.K. Applications of commercial biosensors in clinical, food, environmental, and biothreat/biowarfare analyses. *Anal. Biochem.* **2015**, *478*, 107–120. [CrossRef]
11. Ahmed, M.U.; Hossain, M.M.; Safavieh, M.; Wong, Y.L.; Rahman, I.A.; Zourob, M.; Tamiya, E. Toward the development of smart and low cost point-of-care biosensors based on screen printed electrodes. *Crit. Rev. Biotechnol.* **2016**, *36*, 495–505. [CrossRef]
12. Ronkainen, N.J.; Halsall, H.B.; Heineman, W.R. Electrochemical biosensors. *Chem. Soc. Rev.* **2010**, *39*, 1747–1763. [CrossRef] [PubMed]

13. Arduini, F.; Cinti, S.; Scognamiglio, V.; Moscone, D.; Palleschi, G. How cutting-edge technologies impact the design of electrochemical (bio)sensors for environmental analysis. A review. *Anal. Chim. Acta* **2017**, *959*, 15–42. [CrossRef] [PubMed]
14. Scheiblin, G.; McCulloch, I.; Jurchescu, O.D.; Kymissis, I.; Shinar, R.; Torsi, L.; Aliane, A.; Coppard, R.; Owens, R.M.; Mailley, P.; et al. Fully printed metabolite sensor using organic electrochemical transistor. In Proceedings of the SPIE Organic Photonics + Electronics, Organic Field-Effect Transistors XIV; and Organic Sensors and Bioelectronics VIII, San Diego, CA, USA, 9–13 August 2015.
15. Bariya, M.; Shahpar, Z.; Park, H.; Sun, J.; Jung, Y.; Gao, W.; Nyein, H.Y.Y.; Liaw, T.S.; Tai, L.C.; Ngo, Q.P.; et al. Roll-to-Roll Gravure Printed Electrochemical Sensors for Wearable and Medical Devices. *ACS Nano* **2018**, *12*, 6978–6987. [CrossRef] [PubMed]
16. Jacquemart, R.; Vandersluis, M.; Zhao, M.; Sukhija, K.; Sidhu, N.; Stout, J. A Single-use Strategy to Enable Manufacturing of Affordable Biologics. *Comput. Struct. Biotechnol. J.* **2016**, *14*, 309–318. [CrossRef] [PubMed]
17. Kucherenko, I.S.; Topolnikova, Y.V.; Soldatkin, O.O. Advances in the biosensors for lactate and pyruvate detection for medical applications: A review. *Trends Anal. Chem.* **2019**, *110*, 160–172. [CrossRef]
18. Rassaei, L.; Olthuis, W.; Tsujimura, S.; Sudholter, E.J.; van den Berg, A. Lactate biosensors: Current status and outlook. *Anal. Bioanal. Chem.* **2014**, *406*, 123–137. [CrossRef]
19. Rathee, K.; Dhull, V.; Dhull, R.; Singh, S. Biosensors based on electrochemical lactate detection: A comprehensive review. *Biochem. Biophys. Rep.* **2016**, *5*, 35–54. [CrossRef]
20. Kucherenko, D.Y.; Kucherenko, I.S.; Soldatkin, O.O.; Topolnikova, Y.V.; Dzyadevych, S.V.; Soldatkin, A.P. A highly selective amperometric biosensor array for the simultaneous determination of glutamate, glucose, choline, acetylcholine, lactate and pyruvate. *Bioelectrochemistry* **2019**, *128*, 100–108. [CrossRef]
21. Derbyshire, P.J.; Barr, H.; Davis, F.; Higson, S.P.J. Lactate in human sweat: A critical review of research to the present day. *J. Physiol. Sci.* **2012**, *62*, 429–440. [CrossRef]
22. Boero, C.; Carrara, S.; del Vecchio, G.; Calza, L.; de Micheli, G. Highly sensitive carbon nanotube-based sensing for lactate and glucose monitoring in cell culture. *IEEE Trans. Nanobiosci.* **2011**, *10*, 59–67. [CrossRef]
23. Zagari, F.; Jordan, M.; Stettler, M.; Broly, H.; Wurm, F.M. Lactate metabolism shift in CHO cell culture: The role of mitochondrial oxidative activity. *New Biotechnol.* **2013**, *30*, 238–245. [CrossRef] [PubMed]
24. Diacci, C.; Lee, J.W.; Janson, P.; Dufil, G.; Méhes, G.; Berggren, M.; Simon, D.T.; Stavrinidou, E. Real-Time Monitoring of Glucose Export from Isolated Chloroplasts Using an Organic Electrochemical Transistor. *Adv. Mater.* **2019**, 1900262. [CrossRef]
25. Abellan-Llobregat, A.; Jeerapan, I.; Bandodkar, A.; Vidal, L.; Canals, A.; Wang, J.; Morallon, E. A stretchable and screen-printed electrochemical sensor for glucose determination in human perspiration. *Biosens. Bioelectron.* **2017**, *91*, 885–891. [CrossRef] [PubMed]
26. Hernandez-Ibanez, N.; Garcia-Cruz, L.; Montiel, V.; Foster, C.W.; Banks, C.E.; Iniesta, J. Electrochemical lactate biosensor based upon chitosan/carbon nanotubes modified screen-printed graphite electrodes for the determination of lactate in embryonic cell cultures. *Biosens. Bioelectron.* **2016**, *77*, 1168–1174. [CrossRef]
27. Eikmanns, B.J.; Kleinertz, E.; Liebl, W.; Sahm, H. A family of Corynebacterium glutamicum/Escherichia coli shuttle vectors for cloning, controlled gene expression, and promoter probing. *Gene* **1991**, *102*, 93–98. [CrossRef]
28. Lemoine, A.; Martínez-Iturralde, N.M.; Spann, R.; Neubauer, P.; Junne, S. Response of Corynebacterium glutamicum exposed to oscillating cultivation conditions in a two-and a novel three-compartment scale-down bioreactor. *Biotechnol. Bioeng.* **2015**, *112*, 1220–1231. [CrossRef]
29. Keilhauer, C.; Eggeling, L.; Sahm, H. Isoleucine synthesis in Corynebacterium glutamicum: Molecular analysis of the ilvB-ilvN-ilvC operon. *J. Bacteriol.* **1993**, *175*, 5595–5603. [CrossRef]
30. Ryll, T.; Wagner, R. Improved ion-pair high-performance liquid chromatographic method for the quantification of a wide variety of nucleotides and sugar-nucleotides in animal cells. *J. Chromatogr. B Biomed.* **1991**, *570*, 77–88. [CrossRef]
31. Mosbach, K. Immobilized Enzymes and Cells Part D. In *Methods in Enzymology*; Colowick, S.P., Kaplan, N.O., Eds.; Academic Press: Cambridge, MA, USA, 1988.

32. Weichert, H.; Becker, M. Online glucose-lactate monitoring and control in cell culture and microbial fermentation bioprocesses. *BMC Proc.* **2013**, *7*. [CrossRef]
33. Zhang, A.; Tsang, V.L.; Moore, B.; Shen, V.; Huang, Y.M.; Kshirsagar, R.; Ryll, T. Advanced process monitoring and feedback control to enhance cell culture process production and robustness. *Biotechnol. Bioeng.* **2015**, *112*, 2495–2504. [CrossRef]

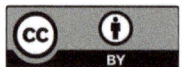

© 2020 by the authors. Licensee MDPI, Basel, Switzerland. This article is an open access article distributed under the terms and conditions of the Creative Commons Attribution (CC BY) license (http://creativecommons.org/licenses/by/4.0/).

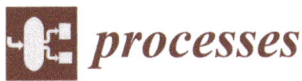

Article

A Chemometric Tool to Monitor and Predict Cell Viability in Filamentous Fungi Bioprocesses Using UV Chromatogram Fingerprints

Philipp Doppler [1,†], **Lukas Veiter** [1,2,†], **Oliver Spadiut** [1], **Christoph Herwig** [1,2,3] and **Vignesh Rajamanickam** [1,*]

1. Institute of Chemical, Envirionmental and Bioscience Engineering, Research Area Biochemical Engineering, TU Wien, Gumpendorfer Strasse 1a, 1060 Vienna, Austria; philipp.doppler@tuwien.ac.at (P.D.); lukas.veiter@tuwien.ac.at (L.V.); oliver.spadiut@tuwien.ac.at (O.S.); christoph.herwig@tuwien.ac.at (C.H.)
2. Competence Center CHASE GmbH, Altenbergerstraße 69, 4040 Linz, Austria
3. Christian Doppler Laboratory for Mechanistic and Physiological Methods for Improved Bioprocesses, TU Wien, Gumpendorfer Straße 1a, 1060 Vienna, Austria
* Correspondence: vignesh.rajamanickam@tuwien.ac.at; Tel.: +43-1-58801-166-496
† Philipp Doppler & Lukas Veiter contributed equally to this work.

Received: 27 March 2020; Accepted: 10 April 2020; Published: 14 April 2020

Abstract: Monitoring process variables in bioprocesses with complex expression systems, such as filamentous fungi, requires a vast number of offline methods or sophisticated inline sensors. In this respect, cell viability is a crucial process variable determining the overall process performance. Thus, fast and precise tools for identification of key process deviations or transitions are needed. However, such reliable monitoring tools are still scarce to date or require sophisticated equipment. In this study, we used the commonly available size exclusion chromatography (SEC) HPLC technique to capture impurity release information in *Penicillium chrysogenum* bioprocesses. We exploited the impurity release information contained in UV chromatograms as fingerprints for development of principal component analysis (PCA) models to descriptively analyze the process trends. Prediction models using well established approaches, such as partial least squares (PLS), orthogonal PLS (OPLS) and principal component regression (PCR), were made to predict the viability with model accuracies of 90% or higher. Furthermore, we demonstrated the platform applicability of our method by monitoring viability in a *Trichoderma reesei* process for cellulase production. We are convinced that this method will not only facilitate monitoring viability of complex bioprocesses but could also be used for enhanced process control with hybrid models in the future.

Keywords: cell viability; prediction; chromatogram fingerprinting; filamentous fungi; *Penicillium chrysogenum*; *Trichoderma reesei* Rut-C30; HPLC-SEC

---

1. Introduction

Bioprocesses are dynamic in nature with varying process conditions rendering inconsistent product quality. Process variability arises from changes in critical process parameters (CPPs) and critical material attributes (CMAs) affecting key performance indicators (KPIs) and critical quality attributes (CQAs) [1]. Therefore, process monitoring is of utmost importance to monitoring and controlling changes in KPIs and CQAs to deliver consistent product quality. Furthermore, complex expression systems, such as filamentous fungi, require cumbersome offline methods (e.g., staining) to monitor process variables (e.g., cell viability [2,3]).

Viable biomass is one of the most important process variables in bioprocesses. Its reliable estimation allows the determination of other essential variables for process understanding, such as growth rates, substrate uptake rates and biomass yield [4]. For filamentous bioprocesses, performance, control strategies and productivity highly depend on cellular aspects, which calls for a segregated view of biomass. The determination of viable biomass concentration via chemical methods such as fluorescence staining using propidium iodide (PI) or fluorescein diacetate (FDA) is accurate but time consuming. PI cannot cross the membrane of living cells and FDA is only hydrolyzed by metabolically active cells, making both stains useful for determining viability. In an industrial setting, chemical analytical methods are not preferred in comparison to physical techniques, which are capable of real time measurement [5]. Thoroughly reviewed methods for measuring viable biomass include dielectric spectroscopy, infrared spectroscopy and fluorescence [6,7]. However, inline sensors are prone to high measurement noise and require chemometric knowledge to establish meaningful measurement techniques. As filamentous organisms tend to develop special morphological forms consisting of compact hyphal aggregation [8,9], process monitoring strategies are further complicated. For *Penicillium chrysogenum* and *Trichoderma reesei* bioprocesses, this special morphology (known as "pellets") featuring dense biomass clumps rather than loose mycelia results in low mixing times and improved gas–liquid mass transfer. But pellet morphology also leads to limitations in the transport of substrates and oxygen [10], which negatively affects biomass growth and productivity. As a result, pellets need to be compact enough to ensure a compact and productive biomass density and small enough to avoid diffusional limitations in the pellet's core. This balance is commonly controlled by optimized agitation conditions, medium composition or spore inoculum levels. If mass transport into the pellet cannot be maintained, the biomass will exhibit hyphal degradation beginning in the pellet's core and a decline in overall viability [11]. Consequently, most contributions dealing with the assessment of viable biomass in filamentous cultivations identify a growth phase and a decline phase. The measurable onset of a viability drop initiates the decline phase. Employing capacitance-based probes growth and decline phases can be differentiated by an increase of conductivity, with error prone results, however [4,5]. Reliable monitoring strategies capable of identifying the onset of a cultivation's decline phase are essential in order to avoid over-feeding and further decline of biomass viability. In this respect, the relationship between substrate availability and oxygen consumption is also a most relevant factor in process control: limiting substrate feeding regimes can positively affect productivity in secondary metabolite production while ensuring high viability due to less substrate oxidation and less oxygen consumption within the pellet [12,13].

Spectroscopic and chromatographic data have been used in combination with statistical models for process monitoring strategies and quantifying process variables. Optical sensors have been widely used to measure and monitor different process variables, such as analyte concentration (e.g., product), product quality attributes (e.g., glycosylation) and cell level responses (e.g., cell sub-populations) [14–17]. FDA promotes the implementation of process analytical technology (PAT) and quality by design (QbD) in each unit operation of a bioprocess to monitor and control critical quality attributes (CQAs) [18,19]. In the biotech industry, such multivariate data analysis (MVDA) techniques are gaining acceptance and are implemented in various leading pharmaceutical companies [20,21]. UV chromatography is one of the most commonly used techniques in various bioanalytical assays. Recently, we employed UV chromatography coupled with chemometric approaches to monitor cell lysis in *Escherichia coli* bioprocesses [22] and for process development of downstream unit operations [23,24]. In a similar approach, we used principal component analysis (PCA) with UV chromatographic data of samples from twelve *P. chrysogenum* bioprocesses to monitor cell viability. In contrast to the previous study, where we used a strong anion exchange monolithic column (CIMac QA, BIA separations, Sloveina), in this study we used a size exclusion chromatography analytical column for better resolution of the protein and nucleic acid profiles. Furthermore, the predictive power of the model was tested using partial least squares (PLS), orthogonal partial least squares (OPLS) and principal component regression (PCR). Based on the model results, the drop in cell viability was identified, and thereby used to define the optimal time point of harvest or measures to maintain high viability through process control; for instance, feeding profiles, power input and dissolved oxygen content [13].

To summarize, in this study we exploit the use of data-driven models (DDM) for bioprocess monitoring in complex expression systems using HPLC fingerprints as a versatile PAT tool. We analyzed cultivation samples using a simple HPLC setup equipped with a SEC column. UV chromatogram fingerprints at 260 nm with statistical models were used to predict and identify the decline of cell viability in *P. chrysogenum* processes. The model results are compared and verified with state-of-the-art viability assessment methods. To show the versatility of the methodology, we implemented the developed workflow for another filamentous fungus strain, *T. reesei* Rut-C30, an industrial workhorse for the production of cellulolytic enzymes [25].

2. Materials and Methods

2.1. Bioreactor Cultivations

2.1.1. Bioreactor Set-Up

P. chrysogenum cultivations were performed either in a Techfors S bioreactor (Infors HT, Bottmingen, Switzerland, with 10 L maximal working volume) or in a DASGIP Mini parallel reactor system (working volume 4 * 2.0 L, Eppendorf, Germany). All *T. reesei* cultivations were performed in the aforementioned Techfors S bioreactor. The stirrer was equipped with three six bladed Rushton turbine impellers, of which two were submersed and one was installed above the maximum liquid level for foam destruction. For supplying pressurized air and oxygen (O_2) Four aeration mass flow controllers (Vögtlin, Aesch, Switzerland) were used. Dissolved oxygen concentration (DO_2) was measured using a dissolved oxygen probe (Hamilton, Bonaduz, Switzerland). pH was measured using a pH probe (Hamilton, Bonaduz, Switzerland). CO_2 and O_2 concentrations in the off-gas were analyzed with an off-gas analyser (M. Müller AG, Egg, Switzerland).

2.1.2. P. Chrysogenum

Samples from *P. chrysogenum* cultivations from both small scale (SS; working volume 2 L) and laboratory scale (LS; working volume 10 L) setups were used for UV chromatographic data acquisition. A total of nine small scale cultivations were tested in a DASGIP Mini parallel reactor system (Eppendorf, Germany), and three lab scale cultivations were tested in a Techfors S bioreactor (Infors HT, Bottmingen, Switzerland). The process profiles for the different scales were similar. In general, the batch was inoculated with approximately $2 \cdot 10^8$ spores·L^{-1}. During batch phase, pH was not controlled. The end of the batch was defined as an increase in pH of 0.5 by convention. After the batch, the broth was diluted with fed-batch medium (15% broth, 85% medium) and fed-batch was started. Details on batch and fed-batch media can be found in [26]. The fed-batch process lasted for approximately 150–170 h. Temperature was maintained at 25 °C and pH was controlled at 6.5 ± 0.1 by addition of 20% (w/v) KOH or 15% (v/v) H_2SO_4, respectively. pH was measured using a pH probe (Hamilton, Bonaduz, Switzerland). After an additional 12 h, nitrogen and phenoxyacetate feeds were started at constant rates (6.5 mL·h^{-1} for nitrogen and 2 mL·h^{-1} for phenoxyacetate).

A feed-forward controller was implemented to maintain a constant specific glucose uptake rate of biomass q_S. Aeration was controlled at 1 vvm in batch and initial fed-batch. Dissolved oxygen concentration was controlled between 40% and 90% during the batch phase and at the set-points 5.0, 22.5 or 40.0% during fed-batch, via adjustment of the gas mix using pressurized air, nitrogen and oxygen. The different q_S and dissolved oxygen values are listed in Appendix A Table A1. The agitation conditions were maintained at 325–700 rpm stirring speed in all process phases.

2.1.3. T. reesei Rut-C30

For testing the versatility of our tool, a cultivation process with another industrially relevant strain *T. reesei* Rut-C30 was done. The optimized media recipe for cultivation has been published elsewhere [27]. In short, the pre-culture medium was supplemented with 10 g·L^{-1} glucose and

1 g·L^{-1} peptone from casein. Batch-medium initially contained 10 g·L^{-1} lactose, 0.5 g·L^{-1} urea, 2 g·L^{-1} (NH$_4$)$_3$SO$_4$, 2 g·L^{-1} KH$_2$PO$_4$, 0.5 g·L^{-1} MgSO$_4$·7H$_2$O and 0.5 g·L^{-1} CaCl$_2$·2H$_2$O mixed with 0.5 L·L^{-1} 0.2 M Na$_2$-HPO$_4$-citric acid buffer (pH 5.0).

Next, a 500 mL pre-culture was inoculated with 5·10^8 spores·L^{-1} equally split in two 1000 mL Erlenmeyer shake flasks. After 24 h at 28 °C and 180 rpm on a rotary shaker (Infors HT, Bottmingen, Switzerland) the pre-culture was transferred to inoculate 4.5 L batch-medium in the reactor. During the whole cultivation, the pH was constantly controlled at 5.0 ± 0.05 by automatic addition of 20% (w/v) KOH or 20% (v/v) H$_2$SO$_4$. Following a drop in the CO$_2$ off-gas signal indicating the end of batch, a fed-batch with (NH$_4$)$_3$SO$_4$ and 200 g·L^{-1} lactose feed was started. The initial specific lactose uptake rate of biomass q$_S$ was set to 0.18 g$_{Lac}$·g$_X$$^{-1}$·h^{-1} and fed isocratic until end of process with an average q$_S$ of 0.05 g$_{Lac}$·g$_X$$^{-1}$·h^{-1}. The broth was held at 28 °C, pressurized at 1 bar and constantly aerated by 1.0 vvm. The stirrer was set to 600 rpm during the batch phase and 900 rpm during fed-batch phase. The dissolved oxygen level was always controlled above 40% by the addition of pure O$_2$ in the gas flow.

2.2. Viability Assays

The following published methods ([11,28]) for viability assessment were used in method development for verification purposes.

2.2.1. P. Chrysogenum

PI Staining

The membrane impermeable dye PI binds to DNA. If subsequently excited at wavelengths of 488 nm, PI will emit in the red spectral section. This characteristic is used for viability assessment according to the following method: Viability is estimated as a ratio between the fluorescence intensity of an untreated sample and a microwaved, and hence non-viable negative control.

To investigate viability via propidium iodide (PI) staining according to [11], 200 µL of sample was diluted 1:5 with phosphate buffered saline (PBS, 8 g·L^{-1} NaCl, 0.2 g·L^{-1} KCl, 1.44 g·L^{-1} and 0.24 g·L^{-1} KH$_2$PO$_4$, see [29]). In addition, 1 mL of sample was diluted 1:5 with PBS and microwave treated by leaving it for 30 s at 940 W in a M510 microwave oven (Philips, Amsterdam, The Netherlands). One milliliter of the microwave-treated sample was used for further investigation. In a next step, duplicates of all samples (including microwave-treated and untreated samples) were centrifuged for 15 min at 500 rpm. 800 µL of supernatant was removed and 800 µL of PBS buffer was added. The pellet was resuspended, and the washing step repeated; 100 µL of the resuspended sample was pipetted into a microtiter well, and 1 µL of 200 µM PI solution (Sigma Aldrich, St. Louis, MO, USA) was added. The PI was prepared by diluting a 20 mM PI stock solution in DMSO, 1:100 in PBS. After an incubation time of 20 min at room temperature in darkness, the measurement was performed in a Tecan well-plate reader (Tecan, Männedorf, Switzerland; ex./em. 535/600 nm). Each sample was measured six times simultaneously using 96 well plates. Viability assessment was subsequently performed according to the following equation:

$$\text{Via} = 1 - (\text{FL\_red}_{native} / \text{FL\_red}_{microwaved}) \quad (1)$$

where Via is the viability, FL_red$_{native}$ is the red fluorescence signal of the untreated sample and FL_red$_{microwaved}$ is the red fluorescence of the microwaved negative control. Viability was measured in six replicates, leading to a maximum error of 5% for each sample.

2.2.2. T. reesei Rut-C30

FDA Staining

Assessment of viability was performed via fluorescein diacetate staining. FDA is a non-fluorescent molecule. Esterase activity in live cells leads to hydrolyzation of FDA, resulting in fluorescent fluorescein [30,31].

For viability staining, 500 µL sample was diluted 1:10 in phosphate-buffered saline (PBS, 8 g·L^{-1} NaCl, 0.2 g·L^{-1} KCl, 1.44 g·L^{-1} and 0.24 g·L^{-1} KH$_2$PO$_4$). In total, 490 µL of this solution was incubated with 10 µL of 12 mM FDA in an acetone solution for 5 min in the dark at room temperature prior to flow cytometry analysis. The calculated viability is the ratio of metabolically active cells to the total number of cells, similar to that described by [28]. Detailed information about the used CytoSense flow cytometer (CytoBuoy, Woerden, Netherlands) is described elsewhere [30,31].

2.3. Data Analysis

2.3.1. Data Acquisition

P. Chrysogenum

Samples from twelve (9 SS and 3 LS) *P. chrysogenum* cultivations were used for acquiring UV chromatographic data through size exclusion chromatography (SEC). UV chromatographic data have been shown to contain process information with respect to nucleic acids (having maximum absorbance at 260 nm) and protein impurities (having maximum absorbance at 280 nm) [23,24]. Significant changes in the impurity release profiles, especially during metabolic stress and viability decline phases, can be used to monitor process performance. The total number of samples from the SS and LS runs were 189 in total. UV chromatographic data at 260 nm were recorded using a modular HPLC device (PATfinder^{TM}) purchased from BIAseparations (Ajdovscina, Slovenia). The setup comprised an autosampler (Knauer Optimas), a pump (Azura P 6.1 L) and a UV detector (Azura MWD 2.1 L). The samples were loaded onto a Tosho TSKgel G3000SWxl size exclusion chromatography (SEC) column purchased from Tosho Bioscience LLC (Tokyo, Japan). A loading buffer with 20 mM potassium phosphate, 150 mM sodium chloride, pH 7.0, was used. The flow velocity was kept constant at 0.75 mL·min^{-1}. All samples were centrifuged and filtered with a 0.22 µm PVDF filter. Random samples (one in every 10 samples) were injected twice to ensure reproducibility and quality of the UV chromatographic data.

T. reesei Rut-C30

The collected samples from *T. reesei* Rut-C30 fed-batch were analyzed using the HPLC Dionex UltiMate 3000 system (Thermo Fisher Scientific, MA, USA) equipped with autosampler, pump and UV detector. The SEC column BioBasic SEC-300 x 4.6 mm (Thermo Fisher Scientific, MA, USA) heated to 30 °C was loaded with 5 µL of centrifuged and 0.22 µm PTFE filtered supernatant and run in isocratic operation mode by 0.3 mL·min^{-1} 20 mM K$_3$PO$_4$, 150 mM NaCl pH 7.0 buffer. Data were acquired at 260 nm by UV detection.

2.3.2. Data Pre-Processing

UV chromatographic data are prone to data misalignments and shifts along the retention time. Therefore, several pre-processing steps are necessary prior to PCA modelling. As described in previous studies [32], we used the optimal correction algorithm to correct misalignments in the raw UV chromatographic data. Three alignment techniques, namely, icoshift [33], peak alignment using fast Fourier transform (PAFFT) and recursive alignment using fast Fourier transform (RAFFT) [34], were screened, and the optimal correction algorithm was chosen as described in [35]. The filamentous fungi cultivations had variations in the estimated viability from the offline analytics; therefore, a smoothing spline method was used to correct offline data prior to predictive models. All UV chromatographic data were scaled and centered prior to establishing predictive models.

2.3.3. Descriptive Analysis (PCA)

PCA is one of the most commonly used chemometric techniques for compressing high volumes of process data (e.g., spectroscopic sensors [36–38]) into few meaningful process features. We used PCA models to identify process trends using UV chromatographic dataset at 260 nm. We chose to use UV chromatographic data at 260 nm, since the nucleic acids have maximal absorbance at 260 nm and can be used for detecting and predicting viability decline. For clarity, we want to capture the differences in the nucleic acid release pattern along the process using UV chromatographic data and chemometric models. In short, PCA is an exploratory technique which decomposes the entire chromatographic dataset to a few latent principal components. In a PCA model with UV chromatographic data, each sample is represented as a score and is projected across different principal components (PCs) based on its similarities or differences. The resulting score plots from the PCA model can be used to identify possible groupings or trends between samples in the UV chromatographic data. The loadings explain the retention time at which variance in the chromatographic data was significant. In general, the first PCs explain most of the variance in the chromatographic dataset. PCA has been widely reviewed for applications in process development and production [37,39,40].

2.3.4. Predictive Analysis

Three different modelling techniques were used for the prediction of viability using UV chromatogram fingerprints at 260 nm; namely, partial least squares (PLS), orthogonal PLS (OPLS) and principle component regression (PCR). The modelling techniques have been well defined and explained in many publications [41–46]. PLS is the most commonly used multivariate method to assess the relationship between a descriptor matrix X and the response matrix Y. PLS is usually used for prediction of quantitative Y data; however, qualitative Y data can be used for discriminant analysis (PLS-DA). OPLS is an extension of the supervised PLS regression. In simple words, OPLS uses information from the Y matrix to decompose the X matrix into blocks of variation correlated and orthogonal to the Y matrix. In PCR, as a first step the UV chromatographic dataset is rendered as a PCA model and the scores from the model are used to predict the viability. The model results were evaluated based on the root mean squared error of estimation (RMSEE) and 7-fold cross validation (RMSEcv). The workflow for data acquisition, pre-processing, descriptive and predictive analysis was applied to the *T. reesei* data to present the versatility of the tool.

2.3.5. Software

Pre-processing of chromatographic data, namely, peak alignment using correction techniques and offline data correction, were done in MATLAB R2019a version 9.6 (Mathworks, MA, USA). PCA, PLS and OPLS models were established in SIMCA v15.0.2 (Umetrics, Umea, Sweden). PCR models were established in Python (using SpyDer version 3.3.6; distributed under the terms of the MIT License).

3. Results

3.1. Data Acquisiton

A total of 189 samples were drawn from small-scale and laboratory oratory scale runs from the *P. chrysogenum* bioprocesses for offline and at-line analyses. Cell viability, biomass, product and substrate concentrations with their respective rates and yields were calculated using standard analytical techniques. An example time course of cell viability measured via PI treatment using a plate reader as explained in Section 2.2.1 from one small-scale and laboratory scale run, is shown in Figure 1. Both runs were conducted at a maximum q_s setpoint of over 0.05 $g_X \cdot g_S^{-1} \cdot h^{-1}$. While the small-scale cultivation's q_s setpoint could not be sustained due to a continuous loss in viability, the laboratory scale run conducted at a high average q_s value was stopped before a massive drop in viability occurred. For comparison, the small-scale run SS4 was conducted at a low q_s at consistently high viability. This emphasizes that lower q_s values help to sustain culture viability, as explained in our previous work: using a design of experiments (DoE) approach, we demonstrated the positive effect of lower q_s setpoints in a reproducible manner [13].

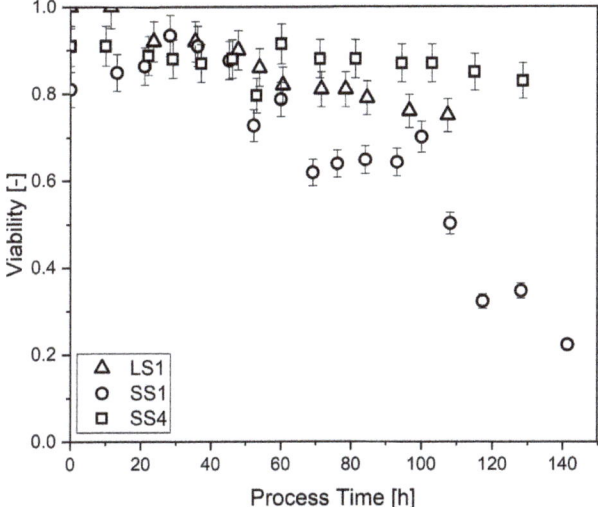

Figure 1. Exemplary drop in viability in *Penicillium chrysogenum* bioprocesses measured via PI staining at prolonged high q_s values in small-scale run 1; laboratory scale run 1 was stopped at the onset of viability decline. For comparison, low q_s values enabled consistently high viability in small-scale run 4.

3.2. Data Pre-Processing

Raw UV chromatograms at 260 nm were acquired using either the modular HPLC setup or a Thermo system with a size exclusion chromatography (SEC) column. Shifts along the retention time in the UV chromatograms as fingerprints were corrected using the PAFFT algorithm [47]. The comparison of the raw data and the pre-processed data is shown in Figure 2.

Peak artefacts and shoulder peaks can be seen in the icoshift and RAFFT algorithms; this is mainly due to aligning the tallest peak from all samples, where the entire data is shifted to give maximum correlation with respect to alignment of the maximum absorbance. It can be inferred from the heatmaps (Figure 2E–H) that PAFFT has removed misalignments, and therefore was chosen for establishing descriptive and predictive models. The offline viability data were corrected to remove noisy measurements using a smoothing spline function. The raw and smoothed viability data are shown in Figure A1.

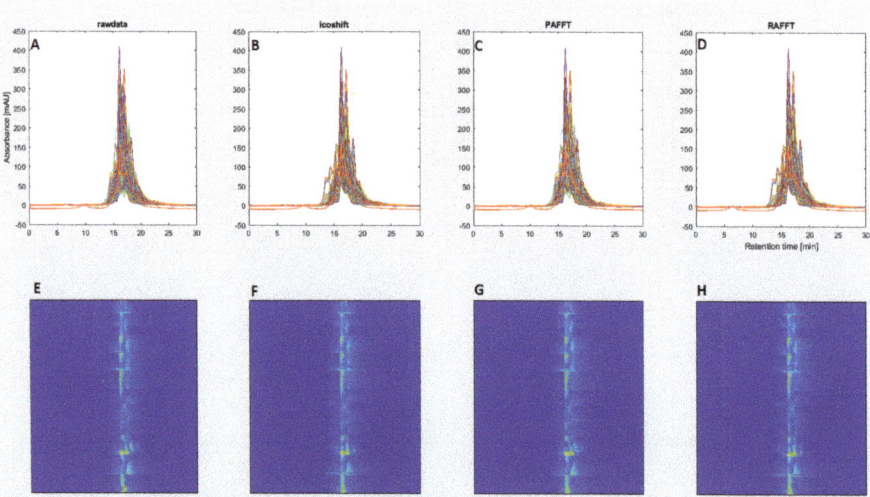

Figure 2. Data alignment correction of UV chromatographic datasets from twelve *P. chrysogenum* cultivations. A, Raw UV data; B, icoshift correction; C, PAFFT correction; D, RAFFT correction; E–H heatmaps of the raw data and correction methods respectively.

3.3. Descriptive Analysis

Descriptive analysis was done as a first step on the UV chromatographic dataset from *P. chrysogenum* processes using PCA models. Three PCA models were developed on (1) the small-scale runs, (2) the laboratory scale runs and (3) the entire dataset to analyze the intrinsic variability between the samples and cultivations. The score plot from the entire dataset is shown in Figure 3.

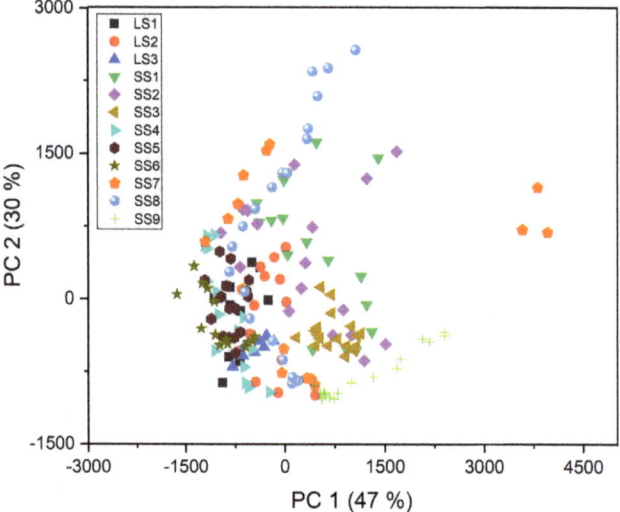

Figure 3. Score plot from the principal component analysis (PCA) model for all 189 samples from the *P. chrysogenum* bioprocesses.

Explained variance from the first six PCs for the entire dataset were 47%, 30%, 10%, 6%, 3% and 2% (adding up to 96%); the remaining PCs were discarded. The PCA model with the entire dataset shows an aggregated cluster at the center of the score plot. The processes, namely, SS 7, 8 and 9 have score spreading upwards and away from the aggregated cluster. It is interesting to note that the aforementioned processes have the lowest viability values (as shown in Figure A1). The scores from the PC2 of the PCA model were plotted across process time, as shown in Figure A2. The scores from the LS runs have a similar trend, since the processes were run under similar conditions; however, huge variability can be seen among the SS runs. We speculate the differences in the feeding regimes, which in turn have dilution effects, caused said high variability in the SS runs. Nevertheless, using descriptive analysis results, a golden batch approach (e.g., using exponentially weighted moving average (EWMA)) can be used to set the standard deviation ranges from run-of-the-mill processes, and significant process deviations can be analyzed. Furthermore, the PCA models were used to detect the outliers from the UV chromatographic datasets based on the distance to model (DmodX) values. All samples which had a DmodX values twice that of Dcrit were removed for further predictive analysis.

3.4. Predictive Analysis

Three predictive modelling techniques, namely, PLS, OPLS and PCR, were used to predict the raw offline viability and the smoothed viability measurements based on the UV chromatographic datasets. The prediction results for both raw and smoothed viability values from the aforementioned modelling techniques for all samples from *P. chrysogenum* cultivations are shown in Figure 4.

Overall, the OPLS models showed best predictive results with an normalized root mean squared error of cross validation (NRMSEcv) of 0.10 and 0.07 for the raw and smoothed viability measurements respectively. It is important to note that irrespective of the scales the model was able to predict cell viability with an accuracy of 90%. The PLS and PCR models showed close prediction accuracy to the OPLS models. The NRMSEcv of the PLS models were 0.11 and 0.08 for the raw and smoothed viability values, and for PCR models they were 0.12 and 0.10 respectively. The NRMSEcv of the two response variables for all models are shown in Appendix A Table A2. The obtained information can be used to detect the onset of a drop in viability and subsequently avoid further decline via adjustment of fermentation parameters, such as the feed rate.

3.5. Tool Versatility

The developed tool and methodology were implemented in *T. reesei* Rut-C30 bioprocesses to test its versatility. The PCA model showed a clear trend with respect to process time, as shown in Appendix A Figure A2. The predictions for the cell viability based on PLS, OPLS and PCR models rendered accurate results, with PLS having an RMSEcv of 0.05, OPLS—0.07 and PCR—0.07. The offline measurements and the predictions from the PLS model over process time are shown in Figure 5.

However, we envision that a robust prediction model could be developed for *T. reesei* processes with higher sample numbers, earlier decline in viability and changing process conditions. The implementation of the workflow showed promising results for this additional organism, highlighting the use of UV chromatographic data from HPLC-SEC for a broader application in filamentous fungi processes.

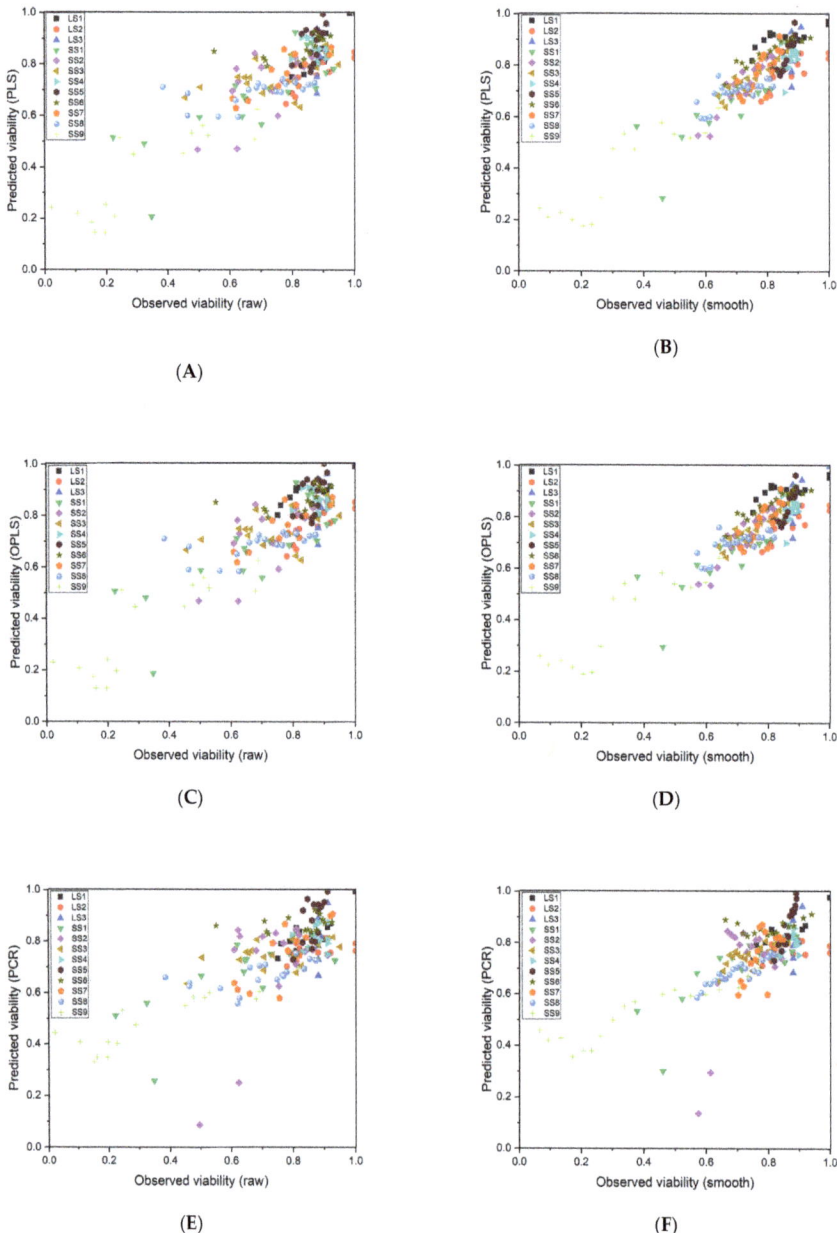

Figure 4. Results from the predictive results of the three chosen modelling techniques for the raw and smoother viability measurements. (**A,C,E**) Observed vs. predicted for raw viability measurements from partial least squares (PLS), orthogonal PLS (OPLS) and principal component regression (PCR) models respectively. (**B,D,F**) observed vs predicted for smoothed viability measurements from PLS, OPLS and PCR models respectively.

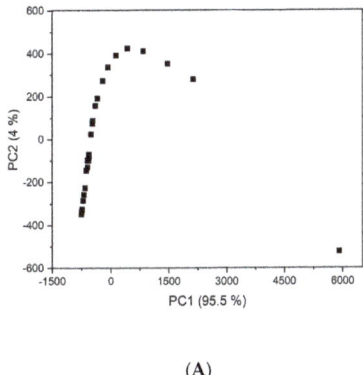 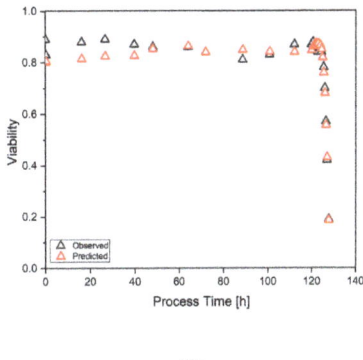

(A) (B)

Figure 5. The results from the descriptive and predictive models for the *Trichoderma reesei* cultivations. (**A**) Score plot of the PCA model, and (**B**) observed and predicted viability values.

4. Discussion and Conclusions

UV chromatographic data have been widely used for process monitoring in upstream cultivations and process development in downstream unit operations. With the rising advances in online liquid handling systems and supervisory data analytical methodologies, UV chromatographic data as fingerprints can be exploited for process monitoring, online state estimation and eventually, process control. In this study, we used UV chromatographic samples from different scales and organisms to descriptively analyze process trends, and using supervised prediction models, predicted the cell viability. Although numerous sophisticated techniques are available based on conductivity, dielectric spectroscopy and RAMAN spectroscopy for prediction of cell viability and monitoring bioprocesses, these techniques require expensive hardware. The HPLC-SEC UV chromatographic data at 260 nm and 280 nm contain information regarding the nucleic acids and protein release profiles from the process. In process optimization, the descriptive analysis can be used to follow process trends and identify potential deviations, especially in pilot scale or large-scale production runs. Numerous statistical methods are available to establish boundaries (usually ± 3 SD with a EWMA), and potential deviations can be monitored and acted upon in a timely fashion.

Diffusional limitations within a fungal pellet primarily involve oxygen and occur in dense biomass structures. However, it was shown that lower substrate availability decreases the consumption of oxygen and can enhance pellet viability [12] as well. Consequently, a decrease in viability of *P. chrysogenum* pellets could be detected and moderated via adjustments of the feeding profile, as previously shown [13]. For this purpose, the chromatographic UV datasets show high predictive power, as reported in the results section.

The descriptive score trends from the LS runs are shown in Figure A2. The OPLS models showed high precision for predicting cell viability, and the methodology has been shown to work for another filamentous fungi process; namely, *T. reesei*. Results from the prediction models from *T. reesei* further highlighted the platform applicability of the presented methodology. Prediction models coupled with online HPLC devices can pave way for predicting the cell viability in real time. Product concentration and potential impurity information can be captured using the HPLC data, and feed-rates can be controlled to boost productivity.

We further envision that supervised classification models could be used to distinguish different phases of the process, and with the use of mechanistic descriptors, hybrid models could be used to simulate the rate of decline in viability and thereby enable process control. All forms of analytical data can be combined to holistically analyze the information gaps in the process, and promising modelling techniques can be used to extract maximal information from such processes. Potential deviations can be encountered early on, and using structured risk-assessment and mitigation tools, the causes for such deviations can be analyzed.

Author Contributions: Conceptualization, C.H., O.S. and V.R.; cultivation, P.D. and L.V.; data analysis, P.D., L.V. and V.R.; writing—original draft preparation, P.D., L.V. and V.R.; writing—review and editing, O.S., C.H., P.D., L.V. and V.R.; visualization, V.R.; supervision, C.H., O.S. and V.R.; funding acquisition, O.S. and C.H. All authors have read and agreed to the published version of the manuscript.

Funding: We thank the Austrian Ministry of Education, Science and Research and the Christian Doppler Laboratory for Mechanistic and Physiological Methods for Improved Bioprocesses for financial support. Further, we thank the TU Wien for funding the doctoral college bioactive. The authors acknowledge TU Wien Bibliothek for financial support through its Open Access Funding by TU Wien. The research article was partly funded in terms of employment (for L.V.) within the framework of Competence Center CHASE GmbH, funded by the Austrian Research Promotion Agency (grant number 868615) as part of the COMET program—Competence Centers for Excellent Technologies by BMVIT, BMDW, the Federal Provinces of Upper Austria and Vienna.

Acknowledgments: Strains for the *P. chrysogenum* experiments were kindly provided by Sandoz GmbH (Kundl, Austria). *T. reesei* Rut-C30 strains were kindly provided by Christian Derntl, TU Wien.

Conflicts of Interest: The authors declare no conflict of interest.

Appendix A

Table A1. The average substrate uptake rates q_s, average dissolved oxygen content and average viability values of the *P. chrysogenum* cultivations from small scale (SS) and large scale (LS) cultivations. Please note that some cultivations were stopped at the onset of a viability decline; therefore, the average viability is relatively high at a comparatively low standard deviation.

Name	Average q_s [$g_s/g_x/h$]	Average Dissolved Oxygen Content [%]	Average Viability [-]
LS1	0.054 ± 0.005	40.0 ± 5.4	0.79 ± 0.05
LS2	0.045 ± 0.004	40.0 ± 5.2	0.82 ± 0.09
LS3	0.017 ± 0.003	40.0 ± 5.1	0.88 ± 0.05
SS1	0.042 ± 0.004	40.0 ± 6.5	0.63 ± 0.24
SS2	0.038 ± 0.003	22.5 ± 4.1	0.68 ± 0.18
SS3	0.015 ± 0.004	05.0 ± 0.5	0.70 ± 0.17
SS4	0.026 ± 0.003	22.5 ± 3.9	0.88 ± 0.06
SS5	0.035 ± 0.003	22.5 ± 6.9	0.87 ± 0.03
SS6	0.018 ± 0.001	5.0 ± 0.5	0.78 ± 0.12
SS7	0.034 ± 0.005	22.5 ± 6.6	0.79 ± 0.06
SS8	0.033 ± 0.005	22.5 ± 5.0	0.78 ± 0.10
SS9	0.040 ± 0.012	5.0 ± 0.5	0.35 ± 0.18

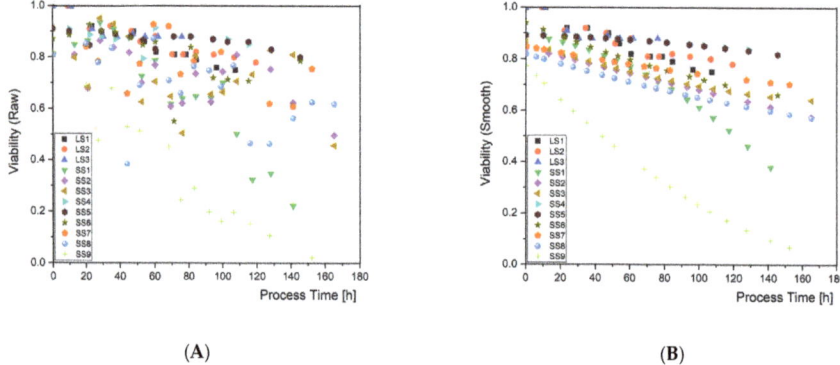

Figure A1. (A) The raw viability and (B) the smoothed viability data from *P. chrysogenum* bioprocesses.

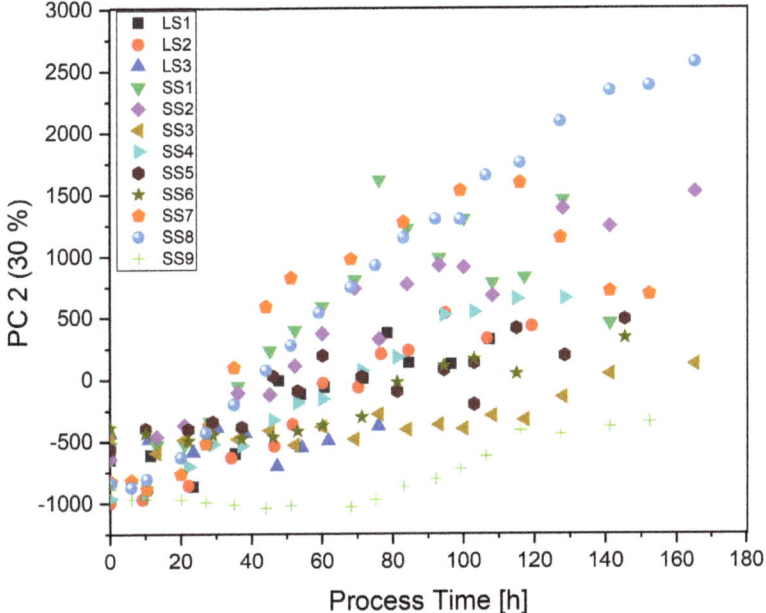

Figure A2. The score trends of the second principal component from the PCA model across process time.

Table A2. The Normalized root mean squared error of cross validation (NRMSEcv) for raw and smoothed viability measurements from the PLS, OPLS and PCR models.

	Raw Viability	Smoothed Viability
PLS	0.11	0.08
OPLS	0.10	0.07
PCR	0.12	0.10

References

1. ICH. *International Conference on Harmonisation Draft Guidance: Q8(R2) Pharmaceutical Development Revision 2*; D.o.H.a.H. Services: Rockville, MD, USA, 2009.
2. Ehgartner, D.; Fricke, J.; Schröder, A.; Herwig, C. At-line determining spore germination of Penicillium chrysogenum bioprocesses in complex media. *Appl. Microbiol. Biotechnol.* **2016**, *100*, 8923–8930. [CrossRef] [PubMed]
3. Veiter, L.; Rajamanickam, V.; Herwig, C. The filamentous fungal pellet-relationship between morphology and productivity. *Appl. Microbiol. Biotechnol.* **2018**, *102*, 2997–3006. [CrossRef] [PubMed]
4. Neves, A.A.; Pereira, D.A.; Vieira, L.M.; Menezes, J.C. Real time monitoring biomass concentration in Streptomyces clavuligerus cultivations with industrial media using a capacitance probe. *J. Biotechnol.* **2000**, *84*, 45–52. [CrossRef]
5. Rønnest, N.P.; Stocks, S.M.; Lantz, A.E.; Gernaey, K.V. Introducing process analytical technology (PAT) in filamentous cultivation process development: Comparison of advanced online sensors for biomass measurement. *J. Ind. Microbiol. Biotechnol.* **2011**, *38*, 1679–1690. [CrossRef]
6. Kiviharju, K.; Salonen, K.; Moilanen, U.; Eerikäinen, T. Biomass measurement online: The performance of in situ measurements and software sensors. *J. Ind. Microbiol. Biotechnol.* **2008**, *35*, 657–665. [CrossRef]
7. Kiviharju, K.; Salonen, K.; Moilanen, U.; Meskanen, E.; Leisola, M.; Eerikäinen, T. On-line biomass measurements in bioreactor cultivations: Comparison study of two on-line probes. *J. Ind. Microbiol. Biotechnol.* **2007**, *34*, 561–566. [CrossRef]

8. Ehgartner, D.; Herwig, C.; Fricke, J. Morphological analysis of the filamentous fungus Penicillium chrysogenum using flow cytometry-the fast alternative to microscopic image analysis. *Appl. Microbiol. Biotechnol.* **2017**, *101*, 7675–7688. [CrossRef]
9. Ehgartner, D.; Sagmeister, P.; Herwig, C.; Wechselberger, P. A novel real-time method to estimate volumetric mass biodensity based on the combination of dielectric spectroscopy and soft-sensors. *J. Chem. Technol. Biotechnol.* **2014**, *90*, 262–272. [CrossRef]
10. Dynesen, J.; Nielsen, J. Surface Hydrophobicity of Aspergillus nidulans Conidiospores and Its Role in Pellet Formation. *Biotechnol. Prog.* **2003**, *19*, 1049–1052. [CrossRef]
11. Ehgartner, D.; Hartmann, T.; Heinzl, S.; Frank, M.; Veiter, L.; Kager, J.; Herwig, C.; Fricke, J. Controlling the specific growth rate via biomass trend regulation in filamentous fungi bioprocesses. *Chem. Eng. Sci.* **2017**, *172*, 32–41. [CrossRef]
12. Bodizs, L.; Titica, M.; Faria, N.; Srinivasan, B.; Dochain, D.; Bonvin, D. Oxygen control for an industrial pilot-scale fed-batch filamentous fungal fermentation. *J. Process. Control.* **2007**, *17*, 595–606. [CrossRef]
13. Veiter, L.; Kager, J.; Herwig, C. Optimal process design space to ensure maximum viability and productivity in Penicillium chrysogenum pellets during fed-batch cultivations through morphological and physiological control. *Microb. Cell Factories* **2020**, *19*, 1–14. [CrossRef] [PubMed]
14. Buckley, K.; Ryder, A.G. Applications of Raman Spectroscopy in Biopharmaceutical Manufacturing: A Short Review. *Appl. Spectrosc.* **2017**, *71*, 1085–1116. [CrossRef] [PubMed]
15. Golabgir, A.; Gutierrez, J.M.; Hefzi, H.; Li, S.; Palsson, B.O.; Herwig, C.; Lewis, N.E. Quantitative feature extraction from the Chinese hamster ovary bioprocess bibliome using a novel meta-analysis workflow. *Biotechnol. Adv.* **2016**, *34*, 621–633. [CrossRef] [PubMed]
16. He, Y.; Friese, O.; Schlittler, M.R.; Wang, Q.; Yang, X.; Bass, L.A.; Jones, M.T. On-line coupling of size exclusion chromatography with mixed-mode liquid chromatography for comprehensive profiling of biopharmaceutical drug product. *J. Chromatogr. A* **2012**, *1262*, 122–129. [CrossRef] [PubMed]
17. Luoma, P.; Golabgir, A.; Brandstetter, M.; Kasberger, J.; Herwig, C. Workflow for multi-analyte bioprocess monitoring demonstrated on inline NIR spectroscopy of P. chrysogenum fermentation. *Anal. Bioanal. Chem.* **2016**, *409*, 797–805. [CrossRef]
18. Rathore, A.S.; Bhambure, R.; Ghare, V. Process analytical technology (PAT) for biopharmaceutical products. *Anal. Bioanal. Chem.* **2010**, *398*, 137–154. [CrossRef]
19. FDA. *Guidance for Industry PAT: A Framework for Innovative Pharmaceutical Development, Manufacuring, and Quality Assurance*; FDA Official Document: Rocksville, MD, USA, 2004; p. 16.
20. Rathore, A.S.; Agarwal, H.; Sharma, A.K.; Pathak, M.; Muthukumar, S. Continuous Processing for Production of Biopharmaceuticals. *Prep. Biochem. Biotechnol.* **2015**, *45*, 836–849. [CrossRef]
21. Rathore, A.S.; Wood, R.; Sharma, A.; Dermawan, S. Case study and application of process analytical technology (PAT) towards bioprocessing: II. Use of ultra-performance liquid chromatography (UPLC) for making real-time pooling decisions for process chromatography. *Biotechnol. Bioeng.* **2008**, *101*, 1366–1374. [CrossRef]
22. Rajamanickam, V.; Wurm, D.; Slouka, C.; Herwig, C.; Spadiut, O. A novel toolbox for E. coli lysis monitoring. *Anal. Bioanal. Chem.* **2016**, *409*, 667–671. [CrossRef]
23. Eggenreich, B.; Rajamanickam, V.; Wurm, D.J.; Fricke, J.; Herwig, C.; Spadiut, O. A combination of HPLC and automated data analysis for monitoring the efficiency of high-pressure homogenization. *Microb. Cell Factories* **2017**, *16*, 134. [CrossRef] [PubMed]
24. Rajamanickam, V.; Krippl, M.; Herwig, C.; Spadiut, O.; Josic, D. An automated data-driven DSP development approach for glycoproteins from yeast. *Electrophor.* **2017**, *38*, 2886–2891. [CrossRef] [PubMed]
25. Peterson, R.; Nevalainen, H. Trichoderma reesei RUT-C30—Thirty years of strain improvement. *Microbiology* **2012**, *158*, 58–68. [CrossRef] [PubMed]
26. Posch, A.E.; Herwig, C. Physiological description of multivariate interdependencies between process parameters, morphology and physiology during fed-batch penicillin production. *Biotechnol. Prog.* **2014**, *30*, 689–699. [CrossRef]
27. Mandels, M.; Andreotti, R. Problems and challenges in the cellulose to cellulase fermentation. *Process Biochem.* **1978**, *13*, 6–13.
28. Lecault, V.; Patel, N.; Thibault, J. Morphological Characterization and Viability Assessment of Trichoderma reesei by Image Analysis. *Biotechnol. Prog.* **2008**, *23*, 734–740. [CrossRef]

29. Ehgartner, D.; Herwig, C.; Neutsch, L. At-line determination of spore inoculum quality in Penicillium chrysogenum bioprocesses. *Appl. Microbiol. Biotechnol.* **2016**, *100*, 5363–5373. [CrossRef]
30. Pekarsky, A.; Veiter, L.; Rajamanickam, V.; Herwig, C.; Grünwald-Gruber, C.; Altmann, F.; Spadiut, O. Production of a recombinant peroxidase in different glyco-engineered Pichia pastoris strains: A morphological and physiological comparison. *Microb. Cell Factories* **2018**, *17*, 183. [CrossRef]
31. Veiter, L.; Herwig, C. The filamentous fungus Penicillium chrysogenum analysed via flow cytometry-a fast and statistically sound insight into morphology and viability. *Appl. Microbiol. Biotechnol.* **2019**, *103*, 6725–6735. [CrossRef]
32. Rajamanickam, V.; Sagmeister, P.; Spadiut, O.; Herwig, C. *Impurity Monitoring as Novel PAT Tool for Continuous Biopharmaceutical Processes, in Repligen Yearly Reports*; Repligen: Waltham, MA, USA, 2018.
33. Tomasi, G.; Savorani, F.; Engelsen, S.B. icoshift: An effective tool for the alignment of chromatographic data. *J. Chromatogr. A* **2011**, *1218*, 7832–7840. [CrossRef]
34. Wong, J.W.H.; Durante, C.; Cartwright, H. Application of Fast Fourier Transform Cross-Correlation for the Alignment of Large Chromatographic and Spectral Datasets. *Anal. Chem.* **2005**, *77*, 5655–5661. [CrossRef] [PubMed]
35. Rajamanickam, V.; Herwig, C.; Spadiut, O. A Generic Workflow for Bioprocess Analytical Data: Screening Alignment Techniques and Analyzing their Effects on Multivariate Modeling. *Biochem. Anal. Biochem.* **2019**, *8*, 1–11.
36. Sales, K.C.; Rosa, F.; Da Cunha, B.R.; Sampaio, P.; Lopes, M.B.; Calado, C. Metabolic profiling of recombinant Escherichia coli cultivations based on high-throughput FT-MIR spectroscopic analysis. *Biotechnol. Prog.* **2016**, *33*, 285–298. [CrossRef] [PubMed]
37. Sampaio, P.; Sales, K.C.; Rosa, F.O.; Lopes, M.B.; Calado, C. High-throughput FTIR-based bioprocess analysis of recombinant cyprosin production. *J. Ind. Microbiol. Biotechnol.* **2016**, *44*, 49–61. [CrossRef]
38. Zavatti, V.; Budman, H.; Legge, R.; Tamer, M. Monitoring of an antigen manufacturing process. *Bioprocess Biosyst. Eng.* **2016**, *39*, 855–869. [CrossRef]
39. Kornecki, M.; Strube, J. Process Analytical Technology for Advanced Process Control in Biologics Manufacturing with the Aid of Macroscopic Kinetic Modeling. *Bioengineering.* **2018**, *5*, 25. [CrossRef]
40. Glassey, J. *Multivariate Data Analysis for Advancing the Interpretation of Bioprocess Measurement and Monitoring Data*; Springer Science and Business Media LLC: Berlin, Germany, 2012; Volume 132, pp. 167–191.
41. Rafferty, C.; Johnson, K.; O'Mahony, J.; Burgoyne, B.; Rea, R.; Balss, K.M. Analysis of chemometric models applied to Raman spectroscopy for monitoring key metabolites of cell culture. *Biotechnol. Prog.* **2020**, e2977. [CrossRef]
42. Chiappini, F.A.; Teglia, C.M.; Forno, Á.G.; Goicoechea, H.C. Modelling of bioprocess non-linear fluorescence data for at-line prediction of etanercept based on artificial neural networks optimized by response surface methodology. *Talanta* **2020**, *210*, 120664. [CrossRef]
43. Zimmerleiter, R.; Kager, J.; Nikzad-Langerodi, R.; Berezhinskiy, V.; Westad, F.; Herwig, C.; Brandstetter, M. Probeless non-invasive near-infrared spectroscopic bioprocess monitoring using microspectrometer technology. *Anal. Bioanal. Chem.* **2019**, *412*, 2103–2109. [CrossRef]
44. Stenlund, H.; Gorzsás, A.; Persson, P.; Sundberg, B.; Trygg, J. Orthogonal Projections to Latent Structures Discriminant Analysis Modeling on in Situ FT-IR Spectral Imaging of Liver Tissue for Identifying Sources of Variability. *Anal. Chem.* **2008**, *80*, 6898–6906. [CrossRef]
45. Narayanan, H.; Luna, M.F.; Von Stosch, M.; Bournazou, M.N.C.; Polotti, G.; Morbidelli, M.; Butté, A.; Sokolov, M. Bioprocessing in the Digital Age: The Role of Process Models. *Biotechnol. J.* **2019**, *15*, e1900172. [CrossRef] [PubMed]
46. Hemmateenejad, B.; Akhond, M.; Samari, F. A comparative study between PCR and PLS in simultaneous spectrophotometric determination of diphenylamine, aniline, and phenol: Effect of wavelength selection. *Spectrochim. Acta Part A Mol. Biomol. Spectrosc.* **2007**, *67*, 958–965. [CrossRef] [PubMed]
47. Vu, T.N.; Laukens, K. Getting Your Peaks in Line: A Review of Alignment Methods for NMR Spectral Data. *Metabolites* **2013**, *3*, 259–276. [CrossRef] [PubMed]

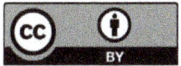

© 2020 by the authors. Licensee MDPI, Basel, Switzerland. This article is an open access article distributed under the terms and conditions of the Creative Commons Attribution (CC BY) license (http://creativecommons.org/licenses/by/4.0/).

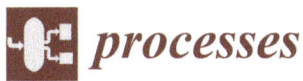

Article

Holographic Imaging of Insect Cell Cultures: Online Non-Invasive Monitoring of Adeno-Associated Virus Production and Cell Concentration

Daniel A. M. Pais [1,2], Paulo R. S. Galrão [1], Anastasiya Kryzhanska [1], Jérémie Barbau [3], Inês A. Isidro [1,2] and Paula M. Alves [1,2,*]

[1] Animal Cell Technology Unit, iBET, Instituto de Biologia Experimental e Tecnológica, Apartado 12, 2780-901 Oeiras, Portugal; dpais@ibet.pt (D.A.M.P.); paulo.galrao@ibet.pt (P.R.S.G.); a.kryzhanska@gmail.com (A.K.); iaisidro@ibet.pt (I.A.I.)
[2] ITQB-NOVA, Instituto de Tecnologia Química e Biológica António Xavier, Universidade Nova de Lisboa, Av. da República, 2780-157 Oeiras, Portugal
[3] OVIZIO Imaging Systems SA/NV, 1180 Brussels, Belgium; jeremie.barbau@ovizio.com
* Correspondence: marques@ibet.pt; Tel.: +351-21-4469416

Received: 31 March 2020; Accepted: 17 April 2020; Published: 22 April 2020

Abstract: The insect cell-baculovirus vector system has become one of the favorite platforms for the expression of viral vectors for vaccination and gene therapy purposes. As it is a lytic system, it is essential to balance maximum recombinant product expression with harvest time, minimizing product exposure to detrimental proteases. With this purpose, new bioprocess monitoring solutions are needed to accurately estimate culture progression. Herein, we used online digital holographic microscopy (DHM) to monitor bioreactor cultures of Sf9 insect cells. Batches of baculovirus-infected Sf9 cells producing recombinant adeno-associated virus (AAV) and non-infected cells were used to evaluate DHM prediction capabilities for viable cell concentration, culture viability and AAV titer. Over 30 cell-related optical attributes were quantified using DHM, followed by a forward stepwise regression to select the most significant ($p < 0.05$) parameters for each variable. We then applied multiple linear regression to obtain models which were able to predict culture variables with root mean squared errors (RMSE) of 7×10^5 cells/mL, 3% for cell viability and 2×10^3 AAV/cell for 3-fold cross-validation. Overall, this work shows that DHM can be implemented for online monitoring of Sf9 concentration and viability, also permitting to monitor product titer, namely AAV, or culture progression in lytic systems, making it a valuable tool to support the time of harvest decision and for the establishment of controlled feeding strategies.

Keywords: AAV-adeno-associated virus; insect cell-baculovirus; cell culture monitoring; digital holographic microscopy; process analytical technology

1. Introduction

After the FDA launched the Process Analytical Technology (PAT) initiative in 2004 [1], an increased effort was put in place by the manufacturers of biological products to comply with PAT requirements. The PAT initiative is a guidance for the pharmaceutical industry for the development of new products and production processes, with the main focuses on: **(i)** increasing product and process knowledge through the identification of the product critical quality attributes and the process parameters affecting it; and **(ii)** monitoring in real-time the identified critical process parameters and the product quality characteristics, ensuring manufacturing robustness and an increased quality assurance to achieve the required levels of compliance [1–3].

Label-free methodologies are preferred, especially in biopharmaceutical processes, since they allow the monitoring of cell culture without adding any compounds which would influence cellular behavior.

Most cell culture monitoring methods employing label-free methodologies are based on spectroscopic techniques, which have been widely used for cell culture process monitoring. Examples include the use of dielectric spectroscopy and turbidimetry/light scattering probes for the determination of cell concentration [4,5], as well as the use of Raman [6,7], infrared [8] and fluorescence [9] spectroscopy, which allow the quantification of metabolites based on direct spectra quantification, but also the indirect determination of cell concentration and product formation based on chemometric analysis.

A label-free alternative to spectroscopic techniques is imaging-based cell culture monitoring. Since cells are mostly transparent, these systems rely on several strategies to generate the needed image contrast [10,11]. One example of an imaging technique with proven demonstrations for live cell imaging is Digital Holographic Microscopy (DHM) [12]. Briefly, DHM provides quantitative phase imaging (QPI), quantifying the phase shift of the light after it has passed through the object of focus, such as cells. This light phase difference is encoded in a hologram which is used to construct high-resolution intensity and quantitative-phase images of the cell while also providing quantitative parameters related with light phase and intensity [11,13]. The way light is scattered after interacting with cells depends on factors such as cell thickness, circularity or intracellular composition [10,11,14,15]. As such, DHM can be used to extract important information from the cell state and has proven useful for several cell-based applications: identification of morphological parameters distinguishing between epithelial and mesenchymal cells [13], detecting cell division in endothelial cells [15] and developing cell proliferation [12] or cytotoxic assays [16]. In particular, infected cells will have different intracellular structure than uninfected cells [3,17,18]. Furthermore, as demonstrated by Ugele and colleagues, DHM-based detection of the intracellular composition of infected erythrocytes even allowed to distinguish between different infection phases in the malaria *P. falciparum* life cycle [17]. The ability to detect infected cells as well as cell concentration and viability makes DHM inherently attractive to monitor the progress of infection-based biopharmaceutical production systems, such as the insect cell-baculovirus system [19].

Insect cells are one of the preferred hosts for viral vector manufacturing for vaccines and gene therapy purposes, since they can be grown in suspension to high cell densities in serum free media [20,21]. However, to maximize product yields it is determinant to infect cells at low cell concentration, to prevent the so-called "cell density effect", a drop on the specific productivity of the cell when infection takes place at a high cell concentration, reviewed in Palomares et al. [22]. The optimal cell concentration for infection and the definition of "low" and "high" cell concentration are dependent on the cell type, culture medium used and recombinant product being expressed [23,24]. Moreover, baculovirus is a lytic virus, which can lead to the release of intracellular proteases into the culture medium, possibly degrading the recombinant product after it has been released into the medium. As such, both culture viability and cell concentration are critical process parameters for this system.

Our group and others have addressed ways to monitor this system using fluorescence [9] or dielectric [3,20,25,26] spectroscopies, as well as using image-based technologies, in particular for measuring the progress of baculovirus infection [27–29]. DHM can go one step further, by monitoring not only the cell diameter increase after baculovirus infection, but also the evolution profile of several cell characteristics, allowing to explore the possibility to observe baculovirus or AAV-induced changes in suspension insect cells in real-time.

In this work, we used the iLine F differential DHM system (DDHM) (Ovizio Imaging Systems SA/NV) for real-time monitoring of a Sf9 culture infected with baculovirus, expressing recombinant adeno-associated virus (AAV) type 2. AAV is widely used as a gene therapy viral vector, due to its lack of known pathogenicity, broad tissue tropism coupled with long-term transgene expression and ability to withstand harsh manufacturing conditions [30]. Estimation of AAV titer in real-time is desirable in order to harvest when its concentration is higher. Moreover, monitoring this system in real-time can support the time of harvest decision, an important process variable to consider giving the lytic nature of the baculovirus and consequential release of proteases to the medium when cells start lysing.

Since DDHM can be used to detect infected cells, we further explored this capability for monitoring the AAV titer in our cultures along with the development of predictive models for viable cell concentration and viability. Using the culture-related morphologic and optical attributes quantified with iLine F, we used forward stepwise regression to find the attributes associated with viable cell concentration, viability and intra and extracellular AAV titer. We validated this approach using leave one batch out (LOBO) and 3-fold cross-validation strategies. As such, we demonstrate that DDHM can be used not only for monitoring Sf9 cell concentration and viability but also for assessing AAV production kinetics in the insect cell system.

2. Materials and Methods

2.1. Cell Line and Culture Medium

Spodoptera frugiperda Sf9 cells were obtained from Thermo Fisher Scientific (No. 11496015) and routinely cultivated in 500 mL glass Erlenmeyer flasks with 50 mL working volume of SF900-II medium (Gibco™), at 27 °C with an agitation rate of 100 rpm in an Innova 44R incubator (orbital motion diameter = 2.54 cm, Eppendorf). Cell concentration and viability were determined using a Cedex HiRes Analyzer (Roche).

2.2. AAV and Baculovirus Infection and Titration

We used the two baculovirus system for AAV production (reviewed in Merten [31]).

The recombinant *Autographa californica* nucleopolyhedrovirus encoding the green fluorescence protein (GFP) transgene under the control of the cytomegalovirus promoter (CMV-GFP) and flanked by AAV2 inverted terminal repeats (ITR) regions was kindly provided by Généthon and was titrated and amplified in house, as described for the *rep/cap* baculovirus (below).

The plasmid containing AAV2 *rep* and *cap* genes was a gift from Robert Kotin (Addgene plasmid #65214) [32]. Recombinant baculovirus was produced using the Bac-to-Bac® Baculovirus Expression System (Invitrogen), according to the manufacturer's instructions. Baculovirus amplification was performed as described elsewhere [9].

Recombinant adeno-associated virus (AAV) intra and extracellular titer was estimated separately using a commercially available sandwich ELISA kit (Progen Biotechnik GmbH), according to the manufacturer's instructions. This kit detects a conformational epitope present in assembled AAV capsids.

2.3. Bioreactor Cultures and Sample Processing

Benchtop 1 L bioreactor runs were performed in BIOSTAT® DCU-3 (Sartorius), equipped with two Rushton turbines. Temperature control (27 °C) was achieved using a water recirculation jacket and gas supply was provided by a ring sparger in the bottom of the vessel. Dissolved oxygen (DO) concentration was kept at 30% by cascade controlling the stirring rate (70–270 rpm) and the N_2/air ratios in a mixture of air and N_2 (0.01 vvm).

Several runs were performed to establish the standard culture progression profile. The iLine F system (Ovizio Imaging Systems SA/NV) was then used to monitor a growth batch and a production (infected) batch, which had similar culture profiles for cell concentration, viability and AAV production titer when compared to previous culture replicates [9]. The growth batch consisted of a Sf9 batch culture monitored until cell death due to nutrient starvation, which occurred after 10 days of culture. The infected batch consisted of a Sf9 culture infected with two baculovirus vectors to express recombinant adeno-associated virus type 2, harvested on day 6 after inoculation. Sf9 cells were inoculated at 0.5×10^6 cells/mL for both reactors. The infected batch was infected 31 h after inoculation, when viable cell concentration reached 1×10^6 cells/mL, with a multiplicity of infection (MOI) of 0.05 plaque forming units per cell, for each baculovirus. The two-baculovirus strategy was used, in which one baculovirus codes for the AAV2 *rep* and *cap* genes and the other provides the GFP transgene flanked by the AAV ITRs.

In the iLine F system, a single-use autoclavable closed-loop tube is inserted into a standard 19 mm bioreactor top port. This sampling tube contains in the other end a cartridge with the imaging chamber.

After sterilization, the sampling tube is connected to a pump motor. Cell culture is continuously aspirated through the sampling tube to the imaging chamber and then returned to the cell culture vessel. The setup is controlled using the *OsOne* software (Ovizio Imaging Systems SA/NV), which controls the sampling rate and image analysis by a holographic microscope. Images are acquired every minute, but image processing occurs in batches of 25, thus yielding a new timepoint every 30 min (the 5 remaining minutes are used for background elimination and attribute calculations). Image processing consists in (1) image focus, (2) holographic fingerprint acquisition for every cell present in the image, (3) computation of 66 image-related attributes for every cell. Figure S1 exemplifies the cell culture and hologram evolution profiles. Acquisition of 25 images for a culture timepoint is presented in Video S1 for the bright field images and Video S2 for the phase images.

Sampling for the determination of reference variables was performed daily for the growth batch and three times per day for the infected batch. At each sampling point, cell concentration and viability were measured using Cedex HiRes Analyzer (Roche). Additionally, for the infected batch, a clarification step was performed (200 g, 10 min, 4 °C) to recover intra and extracellular AAV. Supernatant was subjected to a further clarification step (2000 g, 20 min, 4 °C) and stored at −80 °C for offline analysis. Intracellular AAV was extracted from cell pellets with TNT buffer, consisting of 20 mM Tris-HCl (pH 7.5), 150 mM NaCl, 1% Triton X-100, 10 mM $MgCl_2$ [32], to which a 0.5% solution of sodium deoxycholate was added to further increase the release of intracellular AAV from pelleted cells [33]. After 10 min of incubation at 22 °C, the suspension was centrifuged (2000 g, 20 min, 4 °C) and the supernatant stored at −80 °C for offline analysis.

2.4. Modeling Strategy and Software

2.4.1. Dataset

After run completion, for each timepoint, the average for each attribute was calculated, considering all the cells present in the 25 images acquired per timepoint. This resulted in 499 timepoints for the growth batch and 275 timepoints for the infected batch (online data). These data were smoothed using a moving average of two hours, corresponding to 4 datapoints. The reference data consisted of 14 samples for the growth batch and 23 samples for the infected batch, with determination of the four reference variables (viable cell concentration, viability, extracellular volumetric AAV titer and intracellular specific AAV titer) for each sample. The data for modeling consisted of each one of the reference datapoints time-aligned with the corresponding online datapoints, yielding a matrix of [37 rows × 4 reference variables columns × 66 columns with averaged attributes].

All analyses and modeling were performed in JMP v14 (Statistical Analysis System institute).

Potential outliers in the reference data were identified by a visual inspection of the data time-course profile and confirmed by calculating the jackknife distances for each datapoint. The JMP jackknife outlier identification method relies on estimates of the mean, standard deviation, and correlation matrix that do not include the observation itself.

2.4.2. Attribute Selection and Stepwise Regression

OsOne calculates 66 attributes per each cell. However, due to the high collinearity of some attributes and to prevent model over-fitting [34], the Pearson correlation coefficient was calculated for every attribute pair. For pairs with a high correlation (Pearson correlation coefficient absolute value > 0.95), one of the attributes was excluded from further analysis. This process was iterated until no attribute had a correlation coefficient higher than 0.95 or lower than −0.95, reducing the initial 66 attributes to 30.

For model training, the JMP "Fit model" platform was used. Briefly, the 30 attributes selected were subjected to a forward stepwise regression to find the most significant for the prediction of each of the reference variables. In a forward stepwise regression method, the most significant attribute is identified and added to the model, followed by identification and inclusion in the model of the second most significant attribute and so on. This process was stopped when the next term added was considered not significant (p-value > 0.05).

Since this biological system has non-linear variables, which can be observed on the viable cell concentration and AAV titer profiles, after identification of the most significant attributes for every variable, a second model was created by performing the same forward stepwise regression technique using the significant terms ("main effects") and their interactions and quadratics. The final forward stepwise regression model (main effects only or with interactions) was chosen by comparison of prediction profiles and root mean squared error (RMSE).

2.4.3. Model Training and Validation

Multiple linear regression models were built based on the forward stepwise regression strategy. Two validation strategies were used to assess model prediction capabilities and overfitting: leave one batch out (LOBO) and 3-fold cross-validation (3CV). For LOBO models, the stepwise attribute selection strategy mentioned in the previous section was applied to one batch only. After finding the most significant parameters and determining the model coefficients for each parameter by multiple linear regression, the model was applied to the remaining batch for validation. This strategy was successfully applied to viability models but resulted in significant overfitting for viable cell concentration due to the significant differences in the variable ranges between the two batches. As such, an alternative LOBO strategy was used, in which parameter selection was performed using the reference data from both batches, followed by training of each batch separately. The obtained model was then used for predicting the remaining batch for validation purposes.

For 3CV, the significant parameters were identified by applying forward stepwise regression to the reference data for both batches, followed by multiple linear regression for model fitting using both batches. Model validation was performed by dividing the dataset (37 timepoints) into 3 random partitions, using two for model training with the selected parameters and predicting the third partition. The process was repeated for the two remaining partitions.

The contribution of each parameter to the final model was calculated by dividing the logworth value for each parameter by the sum of the logworth for all parameters (logworth is defined as $-\log_{10}(p\text{-value})$).

RMSEs for calibration (RMSEC) and validation (RMSEV) were calculated for all models (Equation (1)). In Equation (1), $\hat{y}$ represents a vector of model-predicted values and y represents the corresponding reference data; $ncal$ and $nval$ represent the number of samples in the calibration or validation set, respectively; $\max(y)$ and $\min(y)$ refer to the maximum and minimum values for the reference data, respectively. Normalized RMSE (nRMSE) was obtained by dividing the RMSE by the variable range.

The correlation coefficients of calibration and validation were calculated according to Equation (2) using calibration (R^2) or validation (Q^2) data. R^2 is a measure of how well the chosen model fits the calibration data while Q^2 measures how the obtained model fits the validation dataset, which is not used to fit the model, being indicative of the model predictive power for new data. σ^2 represents sample variance.

$$RMSEC = \sqrt{\frac{\sum_{i=1}^{ncal}(\hat{y}-y)^2}{ncal}}. \quad RMSEV = \sqrt{\frac{\sum_{i=1}^{nval}(\hat{y}-y)^2}{nval}}. \quad nRMSE = \frac{RMSE}{\max(y)-\min(y)} \quad (1)$$

$$R^2 = 1 - \frac{RMSEC^2}{\sigma^2}. \quad Q^2 = 1 - \frac{RMSEV^2}{\sigma^2}. \quad (2)$$

3. Results

3.1. Digital Holographic Microscopy Can Be Used for Monitoring Viable Cell Concentration and Viability

Here, we studied the applicability of the iLine F system for monitoring critical process variables in the insect cell-baculovirus system, for the production of recombinant adeno-associated viral vectors (AAV). The critical process variables under analysis were viable cell concentration, cell viability and intra and extracellular AAV titers.

Models were trained using two batches, one infected (AAV production) and one uninfected (cell growth). These have similar viability profiles (Figure 1A), differing only in the time to onset of viability decrease, but are distinct in the viable cell concentration ranges achieved (Figure 1B), as well as the AAV production profiles (Figure 2).

The preferential validation strategy consisted in using one batch for model calibration and the other one as validation set (leave one batch out, LOBO). The high Q^2 obtained for viability (0.72 and 0.92 for validation with growth and infected batches, Figure 1A) supports the feasibility of using iLine F for monitoring viability in this process, even using only one batch for model calibration. The lower Q^2 score obtained for growth batch is mainly due to an underestimation of viability in the growth phase, but the prediction profiles for the death phase (more relevant for this system) are accurate for both runs. For viable cell concentration, the large range difference between runs causes the model to overfit the calibration batch, therefore severely underestimating viable cell concentration when predicting the growth batch, although with the correct viable cell concentration profile (Q^2 = 0.66) and failing to capture the correct trend for the infected batch (Q^2 = 0.34) (Figure 1B).

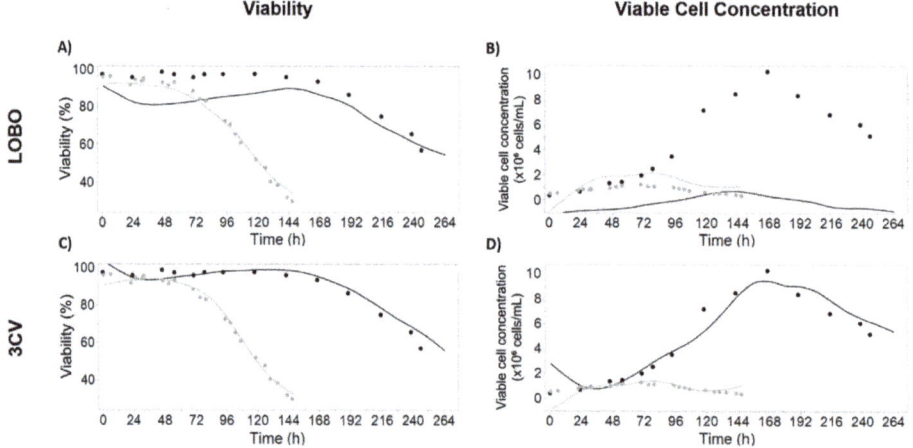

Figure 1. Viability (left) and viable cell concentration (right) predictions using leave one batch out (LOBO, top) and 3-fold cross-validation (3CV, bottom) models. Growth batch is represented in black and infected batch is colored in grey. The lines represent model-predicted values; the filled circles represent reference data; the empty circles were considered outliers and excluded from modeling. For LOBO models, the lines represent the prediction obtained with the model calibrated in the remaining batch. For 3CV models, the lines represent the model built using data from both batches. (**A**) Observed and predicted values for viability using LOBO for model validation; (**B**) Observed and predicted values for viable cell concentration using LOBO for model validation; (**C**) Observed and predicted values for viability using 3CV for model validation; (**D**) Observed and predicted values for viable cell concentration using 3CV for model validation. Model parameters and coefficients are presented in Table S1.

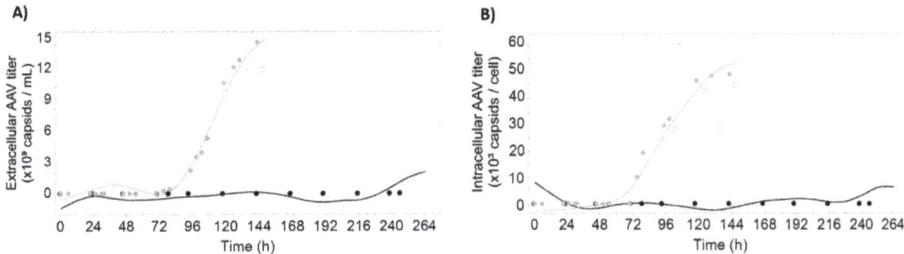

Figure 2. AAV titer predictions for both batches. The growth batch is represented in black and the infected batch is colored in grey. The lines represent model-predicted values; the filled circles represent reference data; the empty circles represent datapoints considered outliers and excluded from modeling. Models were calibrated using the reference data for both batches (filled circles). The prediction data represented by the smooth lines were obtained by applying the model to the real-time differential digital holographic microscopy data. (**A**) Observed and predicted values for extracellular AAV titer; (**B**) observed and predicted values for intracellular specific AAV titer. Model parameters and coefficients are presented in Table S1.

The second validation strategy tested for viability and viable cell concentration was the 3-fold cross-validation (3CV) (Figure 1C,D). Models were built using data from both batches and a 3CV strategy was applied to measure the model predictive power and confirm that these are not overfitting while simultaneously allowing the identification of the most important DDHM attributes for variable prediction.

Applying the 3CV model to iLine F real-time data yields greatly improved predictions when compared with LOBO models (Figure 1, $Q^2 = 0.98$ for viability and $Q^2 = 0.93$ for viable cell concentration). Although less robust, this strategy was necessary so that model coefficients could account for the differences in the variable range between the two batches. The final model parameters and coefficients are presented in Table S1. For comparison purposes, the predictions for viable cell concentration and viability using Ovizio proprietary models are shown in Figure S2. Except for the viable cell concentration LOBO model calibrated in the infected batch, no models consider parameter interactions, since the models containing only the main effects possess an equal or better predictive score than the ones considering interactions and quadratics.

3.2. Prediction of AAV Titers Using Digital Holographic Microscopy

Given that the used dataset consists of two batches, from which only one is expressing AAV, the LOBO strategy cannot be used for modeling AAV-related variables. As such, the 3-fold cross-validation (3CV) strategy described in the previous section was used to calibrate prediction models for extracellular volumetric AAV titer ($Q^2 = 0.97$) and intracellular specific AAV titer ($Q^2 = 0.99$) (Figure 2). The AAV production trend is captured with our modeling strategy, highlighting the potential of using multiple linear regression for identification of the most important optical attributes measured with DDHM and monitoring AAV production profiles in the insect cell system.

To confirm that the obtained models are not overfitting the data, the coefficients of correlation for the calibration and validation set for every partition were calculated for the four variables under study (Table S2). For each variable, the nRMSE for each partition are comparable in magnitude. Moreover, for each partition, the nRMSE values obtained for validation are on average 1.8% higher than the ones obtained for calibration, confirming that the 3CV models are not overfitting the data.

The high adjusted coefficients of correlation for calibration and validation for the models shown in Figures 1 and 2 indicate that good prediction models were obtained, with the exception of the LOBO viable cell concentration model (Figure 3, Table S3). The feasibility of using DDHM for bioprocess monitoring is demonstrated by the acceptable Q^2 (0.74) using LOBO for viability prediction, and by the high cross-validation Q^2 for all variables (0.93 to 0.98). For the LOBO viable cell concentration models, the negative value was obtained when considering the Q^2 for both batches simultaneously, due to the high discrepancy in the variable range and the overfitting in each calibration model. Individual Q^2 are 0.66 for prediction of growth batch and 0.34 for prediction of infected batch. The Q^2 values for 3CV models are very close to the corresponding R^2, demonstrating that the chosen model is appropriate to describe both the calibration data and new datapoints. Altogether, this demonstrates that using only two batches with different AAV production profiles is enough to find the DDHM attributes likely relevant for AAV production.

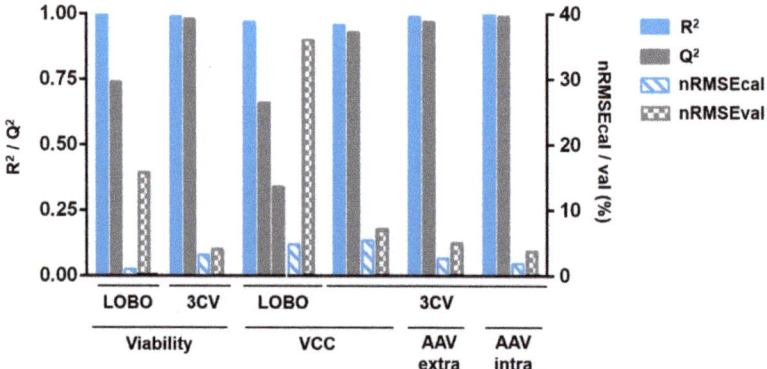

Figure 3. Quality characteristics overview for the models presented in Figure 1 and Figure 2. R^2 and Q^2 are the correlation coefficients of calibration and validation, respectively. Also depicted are the normalized root mean squared errors (nRMSE) for calibration and validation which are scaled by the variable range. For the LOBO viable cell concentration models, the difference in the cell concentration ranges and the fact that the prediction models overfit the calibration batch result in a negative Q^2 (−0.69) when data from both batches are considered. As such, we chose to depict the Q^2 for each batch separately (0.66 for prediction of growth batch and 0.34 for prediction of infected batch). CV—3-fold cross-validation; LOBO—leave one batch out; R^2—correlation coefficient of calibration; nRMSE—normalized root mean squared error; Q^2—correlation coefficient of validation; VCC—viable cell concentration. Raw data are provided in Table S3.

3.3. Time-Course Profiles of Morphological and Optical Parameters Measured with DDHM

One of the advantages of using DDHM for monitoring cell culture processes in real-time is the number of cell and image attributes that are calculated and the possibility to analyze the attribute evolution profile over culture time. While some of these attributes have an obvious biological meaning (for instance "Cell Radius"), most of them do not have a direct biological meaning per se. Still, some of the attributes show an evolution over culture progression and some are clearly correlated with the critical process variables studied in this work, such as culture viability (Figure 4C,E,F), viable cell concentration (Figure 4C,G) and extracellular AAV titer profiles (Figure 4A,B,D). These attributes were included in the final multiple linear regression prediction models with varying contributions for the overall model (Figure 5 and Table S1). Our final models have between 5 and 12 parameters, excluding the intercept term (Figure 5 and Table S2).

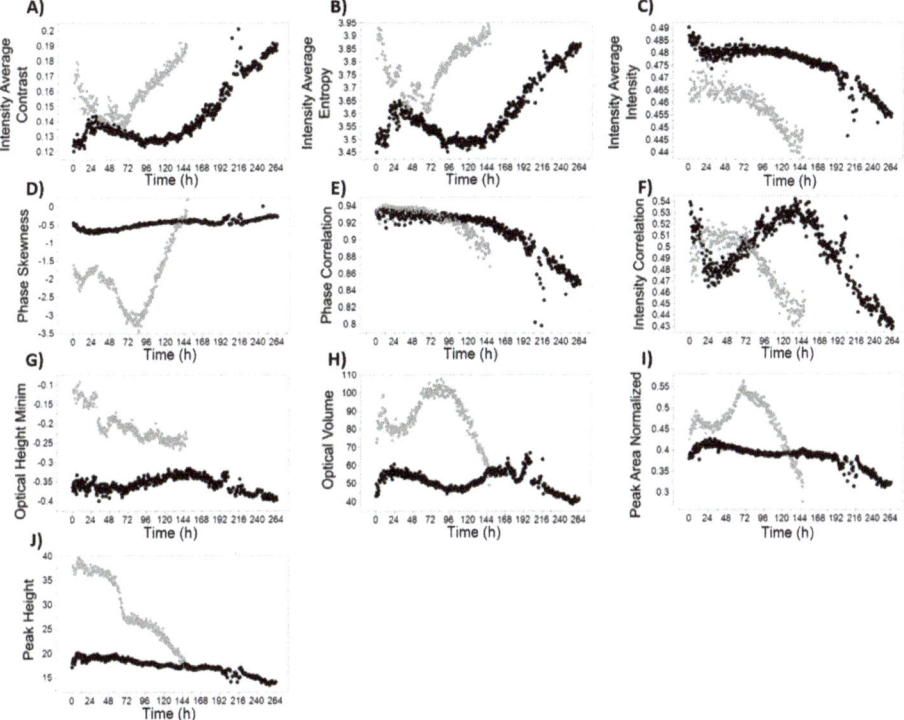

Figure 4. Time-course profiles for selected DDHM attributes. The growth batch is represented in black, while the infected batch is colored in grey. Measurements were obtained every 30 min. (**A**) Intensity Average Contrast; (**B**) Intensity Average Entropy; (**C**) Intensity Average Intensity; (**D**) Phase Skewness; (**E**) Phase Correlation; (**F**) Intensity Correlation; (**G**) Optical Height Minimum; (**H**) Optical Volume; (**I**) Peak Area Normalized; (**J**) Peak Height.

3.4. Model Parameters Have Biological Significance

With iLine F, more than 60 attributes are calculated per cell. These are related with the cell morphology (e.g., "circularity"), the light optical characteristics (e.g., "maximum intensity"), the light phase texture (e.g., "phase skewness") or the light intensity texture (e.g., "intensity correlation"). Overall, the parameters with a larger contribution for the obtained models are related with light intensity and phase characteristics (Figure 5).

Regardless of their relative contribution, some parameters are present in most of the models. Examples include "optical height maximum", "phase average uniformity", "intensity correlation", "intensity average intensity" and "phase skewness". The parameters present in the predictive models for viability, viable cell concentration and AAV extracellular titer are specially interesting because the respective variables are also correlated: viability is the quantitative measurement of the decrease in viable cell concentration, and AAV extracellular titer increase is mostly due to cell lysis [35].

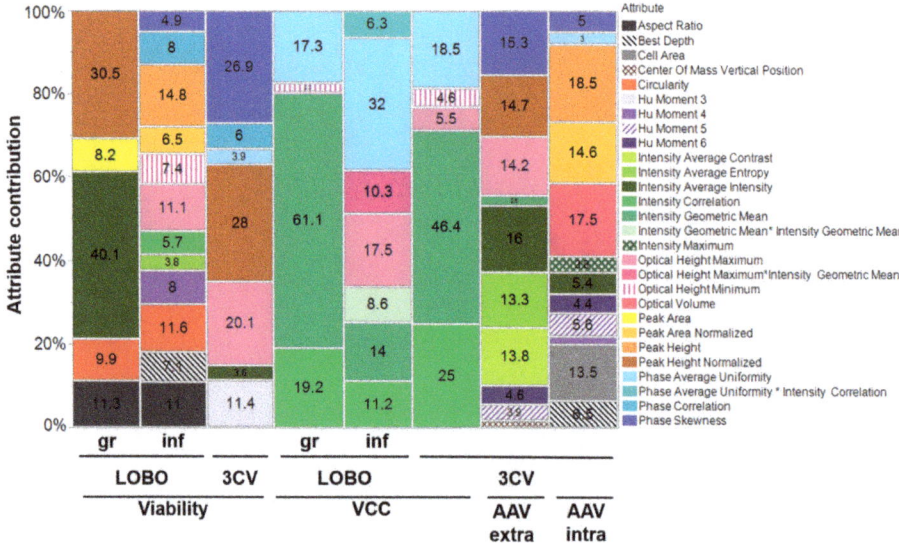

Figure 5. Relative contribution of each parameter to the final models. For the leave one batch out (LOBO) models, the batch used for model calibration is indicated (gr—growth; inf—infected). For the 3CV models, the coefficients presented are related to the model using both batches. Relative importance was calculated using the logworth for each parameter (Table S1).

"Phase skewness" was considered significant for both AAV models, with a total contribution for the overall model of 15% for extracellular AAV and 5% for specific AAV (Figure 5). Although a much higher contribution for the intracellular specific AAV model was expected, the fact that "phase skewness" is also present in some viability models may explain its high contribution for extracellular AAV. As expected, this parameter has negative coefficients for viability models and positive for the extracellular AAV prediction model (Table S1).

Another important consideration is the presence of highly correlated attributes, which may confound biological interpretation of the model contributions. For instance, "phase average uniformity", a measure of the uniformity of the light phase in each cell, is strongly correlated ($R^2 = 0.91$) with "radius variance", the variance of the cell radius, which is inversely correlated with circularity ($R^2 = -0.97$). In conclusion, a cell with an increased "phase average uniformity" has a less spherical shape ($R^2 = -0.88$). The pairwise Pearson correlations for every pair of attributes are shown in Figure S3.

4. Discussion

The aim of this study was to explore the applicability of differential digital holographic microscopy (DDHM) to monitor important process parameters in the insect cell-baculovirus system, including the AAV production kinetics. Specifically, the Ovizio iLine F system was used. A forward stepwise regression technique combined with multiple linear regression was applied to the morphological and physiological attributes quantified by DDHM, successfully identifying candidates relevant for viable cell concentration, viability and intra and extracellular AAV titer.

Currently, there is a lack of methods available for monitoring of viral particles production during cell culture [3]. The existing methods explore chemometrics approaches, by measuring process variables related with the viral production kinetics [9] or changes in the morphological and physiological alterations of the cells [3,36]. In particular, for the baculovirus system, these methods are mostly based on the known increase of cell diameter upon baculovirus infection [27–29], although they were used as an assay rather than for in-culture determination.

Viability is one of the most important process variables to consider in many viral-based systems, being related with product quality and influencing harvest decision [9,36,37]. In both batches, cell viability decreases in the end of the culture. However, the onset of viability decrease occurs with different biological triggers: while in the infected batch cell viability decreases due to baculovirus-induced cell lysis, in the growth batch cells died by nutrient starvation. This validates the applicability of DDHM, but also provides a possible explanation to why the parameters present in each LOBO viability model are different (Figure 5), since the biological reason for the cell death was different. While some of the identified model parameters have a clear similarity with viability profiles (e.g., Figure 4C,E,F); in general, these are not the most important for the viability prediction models. Given the small dataset used, the parameters more important for the models may be in fact distinguishing between infected and growth batch (e.g., Figure 4J, "peak height") followed by fine-tuning using the attributes with the similar viability profile. While addition of more calibration batches would increase the confidence in the determination of the parameters associated with viability, the prediction profiles using LOBO (Figure 1A) show DDHM possess enough predictive power for prediction of viability using only one batch for calibration, and additional batches are expected to further improve the prediction accuracy.

Although the lack of an independent testing set for viable cell concentration and AAV predictions prevents assessment of model validation for new batches, our aim was to explore iLine F applicability to study this production system. Furthermore, the identification and analysis of the parameters correlated with the modeled variables provides valuable biological insights for AAV production in insect cells.

Most of the attributes calculated with DDHM have no biological meaning per se, but can be used to characterize a dynamic phenotype, indicative of the cell adaptation to different biological situations [10,34]. However, some of these parameters may have a possible biological explanation. For instance, "phase correlation", a measure of how neighboring pixels are correlated, has a time-profile very similar to the culture viability profiles (Figure 4E). A possible explanation may be related with the increase in intracellular complexity during baculovirus infection. The cellular phenotype alterations occurring throughout baculovirus infection and the release of intracellular compounds to the culture supernatant during lysis will increase the entropy inside the cell, consequently resulting in less correlation of each pixel with its neighbors and a decrease in the phase correlation profiles. For viable cell concentration, it is expected that the attributes more predictive for viable cell concentration are related to light intensity, due to light dispersion caused by suspension cells, analogous to turbidimetry-based measurements (Figure 5). In fact, one of the parameters common to all three viable cell concentration models is "intensity correlation" (Figure 4F), a measure of how correlated the intensity of one pixel is to the intensity of its neighbors over the cell surface.

Interestingly, "phase skewness" has a time-course profile very similar with extracellular AAV production (Figure 4D) for both batches. We believe this increase in "phase skewness" concomitant with AAV production is due to a combination of several factors: the cell nucleus and nucleolus possess a higher molecular density than surrounding regions, and are likely the cell organelles better detected using QPI due to their higher phase contrast [15]. Additionally, AAV capsid assembly takes place in the nucleolus [38]. We hypothesize that AAV production in the nucleolus of infected cells increases the phase contrast of that nuclear region but not in the surrounding regions, creating an asymmetry. The attribute "phase skewness" measures the lack of symmetry for the phase histogram of the cell and would therefore increase. A similar explanation can be derived for baculovirus, which also assembles in the nucleus [39]. Moreover, infection at low baculovirus multiplicity of infection (MOI) yields a first round of baculovirus release from infected cells, approximately 24 h after infection. The released baculovirus will then infect more insect cells, originating a second round of infection. In the phase skewness profiles shown in Figure 4D, all these phases can be observed, likely validating our hypothesis: first baculovirus infection cycle from 24 h (infection time) to 48 h; and second infection from 48 to 72 hours. The fact that baculovirus and AAV induce a different phase skewness profile (decrease for baculovirus and increase for AAV) may be due to their different shape (rod vs icosahedral, respectively), and the fact that baculovirus nucleocapsid is assembled in another nucleus region, the virogenic stroma [40], among other factors.

Finally, it is important to consider the influence of biological factors such as cell passage or similar. Since we have a small dataset, we cannot be sure whether some of the model parameters are accounting with biological variability between the two runs.

Comparison of the number of parameters in the 3CV models allows to have a sense of the difficulty in measuring the AAV signals when compared to viable cell concentration and viability, which have a more "macroscopic" change. More simple models (with 5 and 7 terms) were enough to describe viable cell concentration and viability, respectively, while for AAV, models with 10 and 12 parameters were needed (for extracellular AAV and intracellular specific AAV, respectively). This is also expected due to the complexity of measuring viral-induced cell changes, in which a combination of methods (measuring nucleus, diameter, cell intracellular complexity) is needed. Another possibility relies in the very different ranges and time profiles for viable cell concentration in the two batches, while for AAV, only one range is available. Higher range variations allow to better discriminate between significant and non-significant attributes. We expect these models to be refined with more batches, excluding parameters which are less relevant and clearly highlighting the attributes relevant for each variable. After identification of the relevant attributes for each quality parameter, it would be interesting to assess how those attributes would change for other production systems, AAV serotypes or packaged transgenes.

Other authors have monitored the insect cell-baculovirus system using real-time monitoring tools, mainly using dielectric spectroscopy [3,9,20,25,26,41]. Compared with other published reports using real-time monitoring in this system, DHM provides a simpler workflow: First, iLine F assembly in the bioreactor is straightforward and no preliminary calibrations are needed; data analysis is in real-time (every 30 min) and immediate (no preprocessing needed) and, in *OsOne*, there is a beta-version algorithm to estimate the percentage of baculovirus-infected cells, which we tried for the infected batch (Figure S2). Further optimization of this algorithm could be helpful to monitor the baculovirus replication kinetics and optimize the production conditions, such as the overall multiplicity of infection to use, and contribute to understanding how this parameter correlates with infection progression. Moreover, the attribute stepwise selection coupled with the multiple linear regression methodology presented in this work has the advantage of generating more interpretable models, when compared with partial least squares (PLS) or other projection-based methods: multiple linear regression models are easier to interpret regarding the biological meaning of each parameter, enabling process understanding under the PAT initiative. This is because in multiple linear regression the coefficients of the parameters itself are analyzed, differing from PLS in which the focus is on the principal components, which are linear combinations of several parameters.

In future experiments using this modeling approach, more "perturbation" batches will be useful to determine an AAV-related "label-free dynamic phenotype" [10], identifying the attributes related with AAV production and gaining insights into their biological meaning. Batches that would strengthen the viable cell concentration model calculations include more "growth only" runs, at different cell seeding densities. For AAV models, examples include runs allowing to decouple AAV production signals from other signals which may be correlated with viable cell concentration or baculovirus production. For instance, infection with empty baculovirus (a baculovirus vector which is devoid of any transgene, but still can infect and replicate in insect cells, and thus generate the normal cytopathic effects expected in this system) or only with the rep-encoding baculovirus. Infection with only the cap-encoding baculovirus would possibly be useful for finding attributes associated with empty or full AAV capsid formation, which, together with the infectivity profile, is one of the most important quality attributes for AAV vectors [31]. Regarding the full to empty ratio, runs using other AAV production systems can also be performed, particularly using systems known by their high full particle ratio, as is the case of the herpes simplex production system [42]. Exploring the application of DHM to other AAV-producing systems, such as the HEK293 transfection system, could elucidate the differences for AAV production in transfection and infection processes and between different producer cells. Moreover, DHM could provide further insight into the reason why suspension-based transfection is less efficient than adherent-transfection. An alternative DHM device with equivalent image processing capabilities, the QMod (also by Ovizio Imaging Systems), could be used to enable a similar approach in adherent cell culture. Finally, combining the DDHM attributes with process data (e.g., DO profiles, total oxygen flow) may further increase prediction capabilities due to the increase of complementary information available [43].

Overall, we demonstrate the suitability of this methodology and DDHM technology for monitoring two of the most important variables for AAV production using insect cells: cell concentration and viability, and with potential for the development of feeding strategies schemes for AAV production. The approach described in this work enables model interpretability, increasing process understanding and allowing to draw conclusions regarding the biological state of the cell at each infection stage. Moreover, models for determination of AAV production were developed, and correlations between DDHM attributes and AAV measurements were determined, identifying for the first-time attributes related with AAV production detectable using phase microscopy. For future work, it would be relevant to employ the same strategy for identification of the DDHM attributes relevant for prediction of AAV infectivity and full to empty ratio, in order to fully explore the potential of this method to optimize AAV titer and quality, in line with the PAT initiative.

Supplementary Materials: The following are available online at http://www.mdpi.com/2227-9717/8/4/487/s1: Table S1: "Estimates, corresponding standard error, t-ratio and logworth/*p*-value for all the models shown in Figures 1 and 2", Table S2: "RMSE for calibration and validation models, scaled for the variable range, using the 3-fold cross-validation strategy", Table S3: "Quality characteristics overview for the models presented in Figure 1 and Figure 2", Figure S1: "Overview of the cell culture evolution profile over time, as captured by OsOne software", Figure S2: "Evolution of the predicted process variables using Ovizio proprietary models", Figure S3: "Pearson correlation coefficients for all attributes", Video S1: "Representative video of the culture at 99h of culture. Shown are the 25 image frames for the bright field images", Video S2: "Representative video of the culture at 99h of culture. Shown are the 25 image frames for the phase images. The images shown in the video correspond to the same ones as for Video S1".

Author Contributions: Conceptualization, D.P., I.A.I. and P.M.A.; Formal analysis, D.P. and I.A.I.; Funding acquisition, P.M.A.; Investigation, D.P., P.R.S.G., A.K. and I.A.I.; Methodology, D.P. and I.A.I.; Resources, J.B.; Supervision, J.B., I.A.I. and P.M.A.; Visualization, D.P., I.A.I. and P.M.A.; Writing—original draft, D.P.; Writing—review and editing, D.P., J.B., I.A.I. and P.M.A. All authors have read and agreed to the published version of the manuscript.

Funding: Financial support for this work was provided by the Portuguese "Fundação para a Ciência e Tecnologia" through individual PhD grant PD/BD/105873/2014. iNOVA4Health Research Unit (LISBOA-01-0145-FEDER-007344), which is cofunded by Fundação para a Ciência e Tecnologia / Ministério da Ciência e do Ensino Superior, through national funds, and by FEDER under the PT2020 Partnership Agreement, is acknowledged.

Acknowledgments: The authors would like to acknowledge Généthon for kindly providing the CMV-GFP baculovirus.

Conflicts of Interest: Jérémie Barbau is an employee of Ovizio Imaging Systems SA/NV. The remaining authors declare no conflicts of interest. The founding sponsors had no role in the design of the study; in the collection, analyses, or interpretation of data; in the writing of the manuscript, and in the decision to publish the results.

Abbreviations

3CV	3-fold cross-validation
AAV	Adeno-associated virus
DDHM	Differential digital holographic imaging
FDA	Food and Drug administration
GFP	Green Fluorescence Protein
ITR	Inverted Terminal Repeat
LOBO	Leave one batch out
PAT	Process analytical technology
Sf9	*Spodoptera frugiperda* cell line
VCC	Viable cell concentration

References

1. US Department of Health and Human Services, Food and Drug Administration. Guidance for Industry PAT—A Framework for Innovative Pharmaceutical Development, Manufacturing and Quality Assurance. 2004. Available online: https://www.fda.gov/media/71012/download (accessed on 15 January 2020).
2. Pais, D.A.M.; Carrondo, M.J.T.; Alves, P.M.; Teixeira, A.P. Towards real-time monitoring of therapeutic protein quality in mammalian cell processes. *Curr. Opin. Biotechnol.* **2014**, *30*, 161–167. [CrossRef] [PubMed]
3. Petiot, E.; Ansorge, S.; Rosa-Calatrava, M.; Kamen, A. Critical phases of viral production processes monitored by capacitance. *J. Biotechnol.* **2016**, *242*, 19–29. [CrossRef] [PubMed]
4. Moore, B.; Sanford, R.; Zhang, A. Case study: The characterization and implementation of dielectric spectroscopy (biocapacitance) for process control in a commercial GMP CHO manufacturing process. *Biotechnol. Prog.* **2019**, *35*. [CrossRef] [PubMed]
5. Loutfi, H.; Pellen, F.; Le Jeune, B.; Lteif, R.; Kallassy, M.; Le Brun, G.; Abboud, M. Real-time monitoring of bacterial growth kinetics in suspensions using laser speckle imaging. *Sci. Rep.* **2020**, *10*, 1–11. [CrossRef] [PubMed]
6. Tulsyan, A.; Wang, T.; Schorner, G.; Khodabandehlou, H.; Coufal, M.; Undey, C. Automatic real-time calibration, assessment, and maintenance of generic Raman models for online monitoring of cell culture processes. *Biotechnol. Bioeng.* **2020**, *117*, 406–416. [CrossRef]
7. Santos, R.M.; Kessler, J.M.; Salou, P.; Menezes, J.C.; Peinado, A. Monitoring mAb cultivations with in-situ raman spectroscopy: The influence of spectral selectivity on calibration models and industrial use as reliable PAT tool. *Biotechnol. Prog.* **2018**, *34*, 659–670. [CrossRef]
8. Zavala-Ortiz, D.A.; Ebel, B.; Li, M.Y.; Barradas-Dermitz, D.M.; Hayward-Jones, P.M.; Aguilar-Uscanga, M.G.; Marc, A.; Guedon, E. Interest of locally weighted regression to overcome nonlinear effects during in situ NIR monitoring of CHO cell culture parameters and antibody glycosylation. *Biotechnol. Prog.* **2019**, 1–10. [CrossRef]
9. Pais, D.A.M.; Portela, R.M.C.; Carrondo, M.J.T.; Isidro, I.A.; Alves, P.M. Enabling PAT in insect cell bioprocesses: In situ monitoring of recombinant adeno-associated virus production by fluorescence spectroscopy. *Biotechnol. Bioeng.* **2019**, *116*, 2803–2814. [CrossRef]
10. Kasprowicz, R.; Suman, R.; O'Toole, P. Characterising live cell behaviour: Traditional label-free and quantitative phase imaging approaches. *Int. J. Biochem. Cell Biol.* **2017**, *84*, 89–95. [CrossRef]
11. Mann, C.J.; Yu, L.; Lo, C.-M.; Kim, M.K. High-resolution quantitative phase-contrast microscopy by digital holography. *Opt. Express* **2005**, *13*, 8693–8698. [CrossRef]
12. Janicke, B.; Kårsnäs, A.; Egelberg, P.; Alm, K. Label-free high temporal resolution assessment of cell proliferation using digital holographic microscopy. *Cytom. Part A* **2017**, *91*, 460–469. [CrossRef] [PubMed]
13. Kamlund, S. Not all Those Who Wander Are Lost: A Study of Cancer Cells by Digital Holographic Imaging, Fluorescence and a Combination Thereof. Ph.D. Thesis, Lund University, Lund, Sweden, 2018.
14. Rapoport, D.H.; Becker, T.; Mamlouk, A.M.; Schicktanz, S.; Kruse, C. A novel validation algorithm allows for automated cell tracking and the extraction of biologically meaningful parameters. *PLoS ONE* **2011**, *6*. [CrossRef]
15. Kemper, B.; Bauwens, A.; Vollmer, A.; Ketelhut, S.; Langehanenberg, P.; Müthing, J.; Karch, H.; von Bally, G. Label-free quantitative cell division monitoring of endothelial cells by digital holographic microscopy. *J. Biomed. Opt.* **2010**, *15*, 036009. [CrossRef] [PubMed]
16. Kühn, J.; Shaffer, E.; Mena, J.; Breton, B.; Parent, J.; Rappaz, B.; Chambon, M.; Emery, Y.; Magistretti, P.; Depeursinge, C.; et al. Label-free cytotoxicity screening assay by digital holographic microscopy. *Assay Drug Dev. Technol.* **2013**, *11*, 101–107. [CrossRef] [PubMed]
17. Ugele, M.; Weniger, M.; Leidenberger, M.; Huang, Y.; Bassler, M.; Friedrich, O.; Kappes, B.; Hayden, O.; Richter, L. Label-free, high-throughput detection of P. falciparum infection in sphered erythrocytes with digital holographic microscopy. *Lab Chip* **2018**, *18*, 1704–1712. [CrossRef] [PubMed]
18. Altschuler, S.J.; Wu, L.F. Cellular Heterogeneity: Do Differences Make a Difference? *Cell* **2010**, *141*, 559–563. [CrossRef]
19. Hidalgo, D.; Paz, E.; Palomares, L.A.; Ramírez, O.T. Real-time imaging reveals unique heterogeneous population features in insect cell cultures. *J. Biotechnol.* **2017**, *259*, 56–62. [CrossRef]

20. Negrete, A.; Esteban, G.; Kotin, R.M. Process optimization of large-scale production of recombinant adeno-associated vectors using dielectric spectroscopy. *Appl. Microbiol. Biotechnol.* **2007**, *76*, 761–772. [CrossRef]
21. Cox, M.M.J. Recombinant protein vaccines produced in insect cells. *Vaccine* **2012**, *30*, 1759–1766. [CrossRef]
22. Palomares, L.; Estrada-Mondaca, S.; Ramirez, O. Principles and Applications of the Insect Cell-Baculovirus Expression Vector System. In *Cell Culture Technology for Pharmaceutical and Cell-Based Therapies*; Ozturk, S.S., Hu, W.-S., Eds.; Taylor & Francis: Milton Park, UK, 2005; pp. 627–692. [CrossRef]
23. Bernal, V.; Carinhas, N.; Yokomizo, A.Y.; Carrondo, M.J.T.; Alves, P.M. Cell density effect in the baculovirus-insect cells system: A quantitative analysis of energetic metabolism. *Biotechnol. Bioeng.* **2009**, *104*, 162–180. [CrossRef]
24. Sequeira, D.P.; Correia, R.; Carrondo, M.J.T.; Roldão, A.; Teixeira, A.P.; Alves, P.M. Combining stable insect cell lines with baculovirus-mediated expression for multi-HA influenza VLP production. *Vaccine* **2018**, *36*, 3112–3123. [CrossRef] [PubMed]
25. Zeiser, A.; Bédard, C.; Voyer, R.; Jardin, B.; Tom, R.; Kamen, A.A. On-line monitoring of the progress of infection in Sf-9 insect cell cultures using relative permittivity measurements. *Biotechnol. Bioeng.* **1999**, *63*, 122–126. [CrossRef]
26. Zeiser, A.; Elias, C.B.; Voyer, R.; Jardin, B.; Kamen, A.A. On-line monitoring of physiological parameters of insect cell cultures during the growth and infection process. *Biotechnol. Prog.* **2000**, *16*, 803–808. [CrossRef] [PubMed]
27. Palomares, L.A.; Pedroza, J.C.; Ramírez, O.T. Cell size as a tool to predict the production of recombinant protein by the insect-cell baculovirus expression system. *Biotechnol. Lett.* **2001**, *23*, 359–364. [CrossRef]
28. Janakiraman, V.; Forrest, W.F.; Chow, B.; Seshagiri, S. A rapid method for estimation of baculovirus titer based on viable cell size. *J. Virol. Methods* **2006**, *132*, 48–58. [CrossRef]
29. Laasfeld, T.; Kopanchuk, S.; Rinken, A. Image-based cell-size estimation for baculovirus quantification. *Biotechniques* **2017**, *63*, 161–168. [CrossRef]
30. Naso, M.F.; Tomkowicz, B.; Perry, W.L.; Strohl, W.R. Adeno-Associated Virus (AAV) as a Vector for Gene Therapy. *BioDrugs* **2017**. [CrossRef]
31. Merten, O. AAV vector production: State of the art developments and remaining challenges. *Cell Gene Ther.* **2016**, 521–551. [CrossRef]
32. Smith, R.H.; Levy, J.R.; Kotin, R.M. A simplified baculovirus-AAV expression vector system coupled with one-step affinity purification yields high-titer rAAV stocks from insect cells. *Mol. Ther.* **2009**, *17*, 1888–1896. [CrossRef]
33. Gray, S.J.; Choi, V.W.; Asokan, A.; Haberman, R.A.; Thomas, J.; Samulski, R.J. Production of Recombinant Adeno-Associated Viral Vectors and Use in In Vitro and In Vivo Administration. *Curr. Protoc. Neurosci.* **2011**, *57*, 4–17. [CrossRef]
34. Feng, Y.; Mitchison, T.J.; Bender, A.; Young, D.W.; Tallarico, J.A. Multi-parameter phenotypic profiling: Using cellular effects to characterize small-molecule compounds. *Nat. Rev. Drug Discov.* **2009**, *8*, 567–578. [CrossRef] [PubMed]
35. Meghrous, J.; Aucoin, M.G.; Jacob, D.; Chahal, P.S.; Arcand, N.; Kamen, A.A. Production of Recombinant Adeno-Associated Viral Vectors Using a Baculovirus / Insect Cell Suspension Culture System: From Shake Flasks to a 20-L Bioreactor. *Biotechnol. Prog.* **2005**, 154–160. [CrossRef] [PubMed]
36. Grein, T.A.; Loewe, D.; Dieken, H.; Salzig, D.; Weidner, T.; Czermak, P. High titer oncolytic measles virus production process by integration of dielectric spectroscopy as online monitoring system. *Biotechnol. Bioeng.* **2018**, *115*, 1186–1194. [CrossRef] [PubMed]
37. Nikolay, A.; Léon, A.; Schwamborn, K.; Genzel, Y.; Reichl, U. Process intensification of EB66® cell cultivations leads to high-yield yellow fever and Zika virus production. *Appl. Microbiol. Biotechnol.* **2018**, *102*, 8725–8737. [CrossRef] [PubMed]
38. Bennett, A.; Mietzsch, M.; Agbandje-mckenna, M. Understanding capsid assembly and genome packaging for adeno-associated viruses. *Future Virol.* **2017**. [CrossRef]
39. Ohkawa, T.; Volkman, L.E.; Welch, M.D. Actin-based motility drives baculovirus transit to the nucleus and cell surface. *J. Cell Biol.* **2010**, *190*, 187–195. [CrossRef] [PubMed]
40. Zhao, S.; He, G.; Yang, Y.; Liang, C. Nucleocapsid assembly of baculoviruses. *Viruses* **2019**, *11*, 595. [CrossRef]

41. Mena, J.; Aucoin, M.; Montes, J.; Chahal, P.; Kamen, A. Improving adeno-associated vector yield in high density insect cell cultures. *J. Gene Med.* **2010**, 157–167. [CrossRef]
42. Merten, O.; Gaillet, B. Viral vectors for gene therapy and gene modification approaches. *Biochem. Eng. J.* **2016**, *108*, 98–115. [CrossRef]
43. Bayer, B.; von Stosch, M.; Melcher, M.; Duerkop, M.; Striedner, G. Soft sensor based on 2D-fluorescence and process data enabling real-time estimation of biomass in Escherichia coli cultivations. *Eng. Life Sci.* **2019**. [CrossRef]

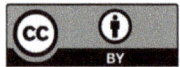

© 2020 by the authors. Licensee MDPI, Basel, Switzerland. This article is an open access article distributed under the terms and conditions of the Creative Commons Attribution (CC BY) license (http://creativecommons.org/licenses/by/4.0/).

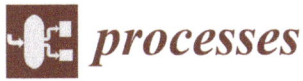

Article

Novel Carbon Dioxide-Based Method for Accurate Determination of pH and pCO$_2$ in Mammalian Cell Culture Processes

Christian Klinger [1,*], Verena Trinkaus [2] and Tobias Wallocha [3]

[1] Roche Diagnostics GmbH Manufacturing Science and Technology, 82377 Penzberg, Germany
[2] Roche Diagnostics GmbH Pharma Technical Development Europe, 82377 Penzberg, Germany; Verena.trinkaus@roche.com
[3] Roche Diagnostics GmbH Pharma Research and Early Development, 82377 Penzberg, Germany; Tobias.wallocha@roche.com
* Correspondence: Christian.klinger@roche.com; Tel.: +49-88566010995

Received: 5 April 2020; Accepted: 23 April 2020; Published: 28 April 2020

Abstract: In mammalian cell culture, especially in pharmaceutical manufacturing, pH is a critical process parameter that has to be controlled as accurately as possible. Not only does pH directly affect cell culture performance, ensuring a comparable pH is also crucial for scaling and transfer of processes. A sample-based offline pH measurement is commonly used to ensure correct bioreactor pH probe signals after sterilization and as a detection measure for drifts of probe signals. However, the sample-based pH offline measurement does not necessarily deliver required accuracy. Offsets between bioreactor pH and sample pH heavily depend on equipment, local procedures and the offline measurement method that is used. This article adequately describes a novel, non-invasive method to determine pH and pCO$_2$ in sterile bioreactors without the need to sample and measure offline. This method utilizes the chemical correlation between carbon dioxide in the gas phase, dissolved carbon dioxide, bicarbonate and dependent proton concentrations that directly affect the pH in carbonate buffered systems. The proposed carbon dioxide-based pH reference method thereby is able to accurately determine the true pH in the bioreactor without the need to sample. The proposed method is independent of scale and bioreactor configuration and does not depend on local procedures that may differ between sites, scales or operators. Applicability of the method for both stainless steel and single use bioreactors is shown. Furthermore, the very same principles are applicable for non-invasive, online pCO$_2$ monitoring.

Keywords: pH; pCO$_2$; off-gas measurement; carbon dioxide; cell culture; reference; cell culture; CHO

1. Introduction

Mammalian cell culture processes in a pharmaceutical environment usually take place in tightly controlled bioreactors to ensure comparable process performance, productivity and product quality. One parameter of particular interest is the pH value, and we agree that there are not necessarily consensus guidelines for best practice in managing pH in cell cultures. Furthermore, reporting standards relating to pH are typically inadequate [1]. This applies especially for publications of both academics and industry impeding efforts to reproduce findings.

The current standard for monitoring and control of bioreactor pH-probe signals in biotechnological processes relies on sample-based offline methods (e.g., pH-meters and connected glass electrodes or blood gas analyzers). Typically, bioreactor pH-probe signals are frequently compared to pH values that are derived by sample-based offline measurement. Additionally, bioreactor probe signals are not considered accurate after sterilization. If the difference exceeds defined criteria, some kind of readjustment strategy is applied, considering the offline value the source of truth. After adjusting the bioreactor pH-probe signal onto the sample-based offline value, bioreactor pH is a representation of the local offline measurement.

Sampling procedures, equipment, sample hold times, shifts in sample temperature and carbon dioxide degassing all invariably add offsets, leading to a different pH in the sample compared to the true pH in the bioreactor. Avoiding those offsets is thereby impossible. Keeping offsets constant between scales or sites is hardly achievable. Especially at higher cell densities, pH must not be considered stable after sampling. Furthermore, offsets must not be considered consistent during a fermentation even if sample hold times are kept comparable because media buffering, pCO_2 contents, and cell densities all change. Furthermore, sample temperatures change after sampling, depending on sample equipment and procedures. Although blood gas analyzers typically maintain 37 °C, this is not necessarily the case if pH meters are used. This also is relevant for calibration procedures that may take place at temperatures differing from sample temperatures. Temperature compensation does thereby not account for temperature dependency of pH in different solutions.

Blood gas analyzers as well as pH-meters are commonly used for offline measurement. pH values derived from blood gas analyzers potentially differ from pH values derived by pH-meters [2]. This also holds true if samples from controlled systems as bioreactors are measured (Figure 1). A sample temperature of 32 ± 2 °C is thereby maintained in all scales to match the at-scale sample temperature if pH-meters are used. Assessing the difference between a certain reference (e.g., bioreactor pH or another pH measurement) reveals a high spread. An offset might be different for the next sample-based offline reading because calibration data, operators, sample properties and so on might have changed between sample time points. The overall information content of a sample-based offline measurement is questionable. Correlations of pH derived by offline measurements to parameters directly affected by pH are often weak or not significant, although process characterization usually proves pH to be a critical process parameter affecting those.

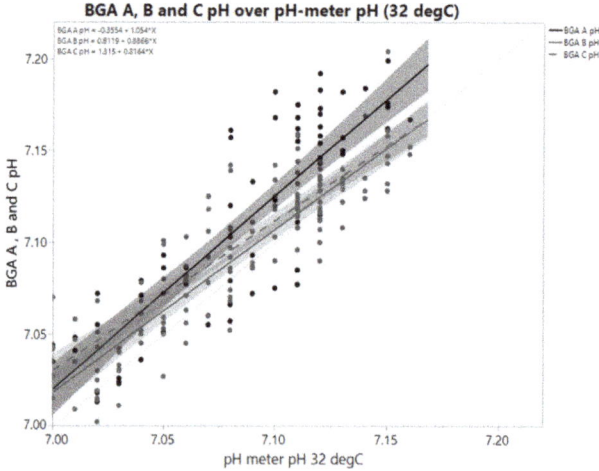

Figure 1. pH values derived by a pH-meter and three blood gas analyzers A, B and C in identical samples; where B and C are two comparable devices. X-axis shows pH-meter value. Sample temperature for pH meter was controlled at 32 °C ± 2 °C. Samples came from eight parallel bioreactor runs (N = 72). Temperature of measurement chamber of all blood gas analyzers was 37 °C. Grey areas are 95% confidence intervals of the linear regression. pH decreases with increasing temperature, so difference between BGA pH and pH-meter cannot be explained by a temperature effect. Slopes and offsets both differ. That means difference depends on either actual pH or sample properties that correlate with pH. Spread of differences is high. A single pH value obviously may not contain required information to justify a readjustment step.

If local procedures introduce different offsets, a pH of 7.00 at one site may simply mean something other than 7.00 at another site. Unknown pH variability thereby manifests in parameters that directly or indirectly depend on pH such as growth, lactate generation, product concentration and certain quality attributes. The amount of base needed to maintain pH obviously directly depends on pH as well, increasing e.g., osmolality.

To enable a more accurate pH control and to ensure more comparable pH values after scaling or transfer of cell culture processes, a method to determine pH without sampling is highly beneficial.

This also holds true when reproducing published findings is not possible due to insufficient description of sampling procedures, equipment, offline measurement methods, sample hold times and readjustment strategies based on that offline measurement. It is insufficient to report a pH set point alone or together with the offline method.

Mammalian cell culture media are usually carbonate buffered. Cells in uncontrolled systems like shake flasks, T-flasks or micro titer plates therefore are typically cultivated in incubators that allow a controlled carbon dioxide concentration to maintain pH values in desired ranges. Depending on the bicarbonate and carbon dioxide concentrations in the gas phase, the corresponding pH can be calculated or predicted using nomograms or respective tables.

The ratios of the respective species, carbon dioxide, carbonic acid and bicarbonate in aqueous solutions as well as resulting pCO_2 and pH, have been published in satisfactory detail elsewhere and are usually part of academic training [3,4]. It is very important to note that not only pH and carbon dioxide in the gas phase must correlate. Since carbon dioxide in the gas phase and dissolved carbon dioxide are directly related via the same chemical principles, we also must be able to estimate dissolved carbon dioxide (pCO_2) with off-gas analysis. However, to match sample-based offline pCO_2 values and the actual pCO_2 in the bioreactor, sample hold times had to be included as well due to changes in carbon dioxide concentration in closed sample containers after sampling before measurement. This means that like pH, pCO_2 derived by sample-based offline measurement may not be representative of the true value in bioreactors, partly via the very same mechanisms like carbon dioxide degassing during the sampling process or carbon dioxide accumulation via respiration. The potential to estimate pCO_2 levels and trends via off-gas analysis is also discussed in this paper very briefly.

Interrelations between pH, pCO_2, bicarbonate and dissolved carbon dioxide are not dependent on scale or, e.g., bioreactor configuration. pH will be identical in identical medium at a given carbon dioxide concentration in the gas phase no matter what volume a given shake flask has, or if that is compared to the pH in a T-flask in the same incubator. This is true in any system including bioreactors, where carbon dioxide is used as an acidic component for pH control, counteracting any carbon dioxide removal by aeration of this bioreactor.

We can assume that in equilibrium, flux of exhaust carbon dioxide equals carbon dioxide influx. Under this assumption, overall CO_2 mass in the bioreactor must be constant. Given constant pressure and temperature, dissolved carbon dioxide and bicarbonate concentration and pH must be constant as well.

This means pH in a given cell culture medium can be calculated if carbon dioxide concentration in a respective bioreactor gas phase is known, and if both carbon dioxide concentration and pH are kept stable, e.g., via pH control or defined gas influx containing carbon dioxide. This is also true not only for stainless steel bioreactors, but also for single use bioreactors. Technical implementation of off-gas analysis itself might differ depending on the bioreactor used, but underlying principles stay the same [5]. The correlation of pH and corresponding carbon dioxide concentration in the gas phase is thereby universal and applicable, independent of location and the vessel used.

Nonetheless, in GMP manufacturing the independence of this method from scale and bioreactor configuration has to be proven and validated against the standard established method, which is sample-based offline measurement. As described, sample-based offline pH measurement comes with inherent variability. To validate the off-gas-based pH reference method, we still have to refer to the very same sample-based offline measurement that we want to replace by a more accurate method.

An unintended shift in pH after changing to the proposed method in legacy products therefore needs to be avoided. The proposed method is able to determine the true pH in the bioreactor without sampling and offsets introduced by the sample-based offline method. On the other hand, we are currently using sample-based offline measurement to monitor and readjust our bioreactor pH-probes. Offsets currently introduced by sample-based offline measurement must therefore be accurately determined. Either pH set points have to be adapted to match the true pH, or the offsets have to be incorporated in the method itself.

In 2004, the U.S. Department of Health and Human Services Food and Drug Administration published a framework for Innovative Pharmaceutical Development, Manufacturing, and Quality Assurance, emphasizing the need for applying scientific and engineering principles to ensure acceptable and reproducible product quality in manufacturing processes. Thereby, pH must be considered a relevant parameter affecting product quality and overall process performance in mammalian cell culture. Any significant advance in the ability to get this parameter better and more accurately controlled might have a positive impact on overall process control and in the end patient safety.

Furthermore, reproducing findings that have been achieved somewhere else in the scientific community would finally be possible as well in the field of mammalian cell culture where different cell lines, proprietary media and insufficient description of materials and methods slow down potential overall progress.

2. Materials and Methods

2.1. Determination of Media Specific Correlations of the pH and Corresponding Exhaust Carbon Dioxide Concentration

To determine the exhaust carbon dioxide concentration, an off-gas measurement was established (DASGIP® GA4 (Eppendorf AG, Hamburg, Germany). Carbon dioxide concentration was determined with double beam infrared absorption. Pressure compensation was inactive; environmental pressure was set to 941 mbar (Roche Site in Penzberg is 621 m in height). The CO_2 sensor was two point calibrated before use with process air and a defined gas mixture (Linde AG) containing 24% CO_2 and 2% O_2.

Two-Liter Bioreactors (Sartorius B-DCU Quad) with a total volume of 3 L and typical working volumes of around 2 L were connected to the off-gas sensors with gas tight tubing. For experimental determination of media specific correlations of pH and a corresponding exhaust carbon dioxide concentration up to 2.5 L, medium was used to minimize headspace volume. Pressure control valve, sterile filter and exhaust cooling at around ten °C were integrated in the exhaust line. Pressure was controlled to match at-scale total pressures for respective products. Bioreactors and pH probes (Mettler Toledo, InPro3253/225/PT100) were sterilized wet in 1.2 g/L $KH_2PO_{4(aq)}$. Media fill was performed under sterile conditions.

Bioreactor pH was determined with a built in online-pH probe that was initially two point calibrated in buffers (4.00 and 7.00 at 25 °C, Mettler Toledo). Carbon dioxide gas was used as an acidic pH correction agent via pH control to maintain pH at upper dead bands. The pH controller was set up as a proportional controller to achieve a constant carbon dioxide influx. No basic correction agent was used, and so pH thereby naturally increases by carbon dioxide removal via constant aeration with process air.

After sterilization and media fill a hold step to stabilize pH, pressure and temperature were established. To enable accurate pH readings, a port in the bioreactor lid was opened, making the system unsterile in the process. Two independent pH-probes (Mettler Toledo InLab Semi-Micro) connected to respective pH-meters (Knick Portavo 907) were inserted simultaneously through the open port into the bioreactor to measure pH in the liquid phase without sampling. Agitation, aeration and temperature control all stayed active. Pressure control was set to inactive. pH-meters were independently three point calibrated (Mettler Toledo buffers 9.21, 7.00, 4.00 at 25 °C) with active automated temperature compensation (ATC). The average of the pH-meter readings was used to standardize (one point adjustment) the online bioreactor pH probe signal. Maximum acceptable difference of the pH meter signals was thereby 0.02, and the maximum difference from the buffer pH was 0.01. The same procedure was performed to check bioreactor pH after the experiment again to detect any unintended drifts of the bioreactor probe signal.

After standardization of the bioreactor probe signal, the bioreactor lid was closed again and pressure control was set as active. After establishing an equilibrium (stable pH and carbon dioxide concentration in the exhaust gas) the first data point online pH and corresponding exhaust carbon dioxide concentration was documented. Correlations were determined in four technical replicates, which means four independent bioreactors filled with identical medium. Four pH set points were determined in each bioreactor. After establishing an equilibrium at every set point, pH was also determined via a sample-based offline measurement (Sarstedt Monovette, Knick Portavo 970 with connected Mettler Toledo InLab Semi-Micro Pro pH probe). Sample temperature thereby was kept at $32 \pm 2\ °C$ using appropriate sample tempering.

The cell culture medium shown in this paper is a bicarbonate buffered, complex proprietary medium.

2.2. Transfer and Use of Correlations in GMP Manufacturing

Correlations were fitted with quadratic regression (JMP 12). For transfer purposes, the equation was transferred to a new plant or site. All bioreactors in GMP manufacturing or clinical plants were equipped with two redundant, independent pH probes. Readjustment of bioreactor probes after media fill before inoculation was based on the result of this equation after actual carbon dioxide concentration was fed into the equation. The calculated pH was then used to initially standardize respective bioreactor probe signals. To detect potential bioreactor pH probe signal drifts, the readjustment strategy was adjusted to rely on delta probe alarms as a detection measure instead of frequent sample-based offline readings. Readjustments based on sample-based offline measurements only took place if a justified suspicion for a double probe drift that is not detectable by a delta probe alarm did exist. In case of a single probe drift detectable by a delta probe alarm an offline reading was utilized to determine which one of the probes measured incorrectly. A readjustment onto the offline value was thereby avoided at all times.

To establish an accurate reading, the carbonate buffered medium in the bioreactor has to be in equilibrium with its gas phase, which means either the pH control adds as much carbon dioxide as is removed via aeration or a defined influx containing carbon dioxide is used leading to stable readings of pH and corresponding carbon dioxide in both cases. Depending on scale and the ratio between headspace and working volume, the time until equilibrium may take more time then feasible. Aeration rates were adapted in those cases to accelerate headspace back mixing.

Additional parameters potentially adding errors like overpressure, headspace aeration, exhaust humidity and condensate, overall gas flow rates and so on were kept identical or adapted accordingly.

2.3. Validation of Scale Independency and Offset Determination to Established Sample-Based Offline Measurement

To prove independence of scale in an established commercial process, a correlation pH and corresponding exhaust carbon dioxide concentration were determined on a small scale as described above. Scale independency was proven by using the very same correlation in another scale (20 L) to adjust the bioreactor probe signal onto a calculated pH based on this correlation. After adjustment, the bioreactor was again made unsterile to directly measure with accurately calibrated pH-meters in the liquid phase of that bioreactor to prove the true pH to be comparable given the defined acceptance criteria.

To prove that the proposed method is as good or better as the established sample-based offline pH in scale up to 5k, pH values were calculated for each scale for the respective product using the quadratic fit for the media specific correlation. Equivalence of the offsets between sample-based offline values and the calculated pH was then tested using a two-sided student's t-test (TOST). As practically significant differences (PSDs), the double standard deviation of historic differences of sample-based offline measurement and bioreactor pH was calculated. Equivalence is thereby considered proof that sample-based offline measurement does not generate different offsets on different scales due to different procedures and equipment.

2.4. Influence of pH Correction Agents Added during Media Preparation

Media preparation was considered with respect to weighing and dosing tolerances. pH correction agents especially directly affect the correlation pH and corresponding carbon dioxide concentration in consecutive bioreactors where those media are used. The lower the lot-to-lot variability is, the higher the accuracy of the carbon dioxide-based pH reference method will be.

Respective cell culture medium was filled in bioreactors (Sartorius B-DCU Quad). pH control was set as active, and no basic solution attached. The aeration rate was set constant to 50 ccm. After reaching equilibrium, where pH is maintained at the upper dead band by a constant carbon dioxide influx applied by pH control, the first data point pH and corresponding exhaust carbon dioxide concentration were documented. After adding a defined amount of pH correction agent, the next data point pH and corresponding exhaust carbon dioxide concentration were documented. Two technical replicates were used for two media lots to determine the difference in exhaust carbon dioxide readings at identical bioreactor pH caused by base addition.

Generally, for comparable media, comparable amounts of pH correction agent should be required. If media pH is adjusted to desired pH levels based on pH readings generated in the very same media by varying amounts of pH correction agents, conditions in bioreactors filled with those media cannot be achieved because the pH controller response, such as adding base and acid, will be altered. Furthermore, the very important process control (pH in finished medium) is annulled if media pH is adjusted because pH will always be in range after adjustment.

All projects so far that utilized the proposed method internally implemented fixed amounts of pH correction agents.

2.5. Exhaust Gas Analysis in Single Use Bioreactors (SUBs)

To determine carbon dioxide concentration in the exhaust gas of SUBs, DASGIP® GA4 (Eppendorf AG, Hamburg, Germany) devices were used. Before use, sensors were two point calibrated with process air and a defined gas mixture (Linde AG) containing 2% oxygen, 10% carbon dioxide (up to 250 L non GMP runs) and 24% carbon dioxide (2K GMP runs), respectively, to ensure a stable gas composition measurement at given ambient conditions. A membrane pump was connected after respective exhaust filters to ensure a stable and pulsation free exhaust gas flux from 250 L and 2k single use bioreactors w/o pressure control. Exhaust filter-heating prevented blocking. Condensate traps in the exhaust line removed any condensate generated by cooling of the saturated exhaust gas stream after filters.

All Ambr250™ multi fermenter systems (Sartorius Stedim Biotech AG, Göttingen, Germany) have a built-in off-gas analyzer module to measure O_2 and CO_2 in the exhaust flow of all 12 bioreactor vessels simultaneously with sufficient accuracy. CO_2 sensors in Ambr250 were five-point calibrated with different defined gas mixtures (Linde AG) to reach calibration points at 0%, 3%, 5%, 8% and 16% CO_2.

In all runs performed in SUBs, recombinant CHO suspension cell lines expressing different types of antibodies were cultivated in one culture medium (proprietary chemically defined Roche medium).

For standardization of the bioreactor pH-probe signal, respective media was subsequently equilibrated with a defined gas mixture (93% process air and 7% CO_2) after media fill until saturation. After equilibration phase, culture pH was calculated from the exhaust carbon dioxide concentration in all scales based on the calibration function according to the described method above. Bioreactor probe signal was then adjusted onto the calculated pH.

Sample-based offline measurement was performed with varying methods depending on vessel size. Ambr250™ built-in analysis module was two point calibrated (Sartorius Stedim buffers 4.00, 7.00 at 25 °C). A liquid handling system (200 µL) did perform sampling and offline pH measurement.

On the 250 L SUB scale, samples were drawn using a sterile syringe and pH was offline measured by a calibrated (Nova Biomedical calibration cartridge) blood gas analyzer (BioProfile® pHOx® Analyzer, Nova Biomedical GmbH, Mörfelden-Walldorf, Germany).

Samples in 2k SUBs in a GMP environment were also drawn using a sterile syringe and transferred into a preheated falcon tube. Offline pH was measured by a two point adjusted glass electrode (Knick Portavo 970 with connected Mettler Toledo Semi Micro pH probe, Mettler Toledo buffers 7.00, 4.00 at 25 °C).

2.6. Exhaust Gas Analysis for Monitoring of Dissolved Carbon Dioxide

A recombinant CHO clone (Chinese Hamster Ovary cells, suspension culture) constitutively expressing an antibody was cultivated in proprietary chemically-defined cell culture media. All cell cultivations used for calibration of the pCO_2 model took place in a 2 L stirred tank bioreactor (BIOSTAT® B-DCU Quad, Sartorius, Göttingen) for approximately 14 days cultivation time. Temperature, DO, pressure and pH were all controlled and kept constant for all runs shown.

Daily sample-based offline pCO_2 measurement samples were drawn using a closed and tempered (32 °C ± 2 °C, Sarstedt Monovette) container to minimize unintended carbon dioxide. pCO_2 was determined by a blood gas analyzer (cobas b 221, Roche Custom Biotech Mannheim, Germany).

Exhaust carbon dioxide concentration again was determined as described above (DASGIP® GA4 (Eppendorf AG, Hamburg, Germany).

The data set for developing a suitable model included a total of 32 cell cultivations. Calculations and modelling was carried out using JMP 12 (SAS, Cary, NC, USA) and Microsoft Excel 2016 (Redmond, WA, USA). The data set was split into a calibration set, containing 24 of the runs, and an external validation set comprising the remaining runs (1/4 of the complete data set). The model contained the actual exhaust carbon dioxide concentration as a quadratic effect, and actual pH, as equilibrium constants of the carbonate buffer systems depend on pH [4] and sample hold times to account for carbon dioxide changes in the sample until measurement. Those changes can easily be detected by calculating the ratio of pCO_2 and exhaust carbon dioxide concentration. Exhaust carbon dioxide concentration does not change by sampling, whereas pCO_2 in the sample does change. Looking at the ratio allows one to detect pCO_2 changes in a sample by simply plotting it against a sample hold time, whereas measuring multiple times in one sample would potentially affect the outcome. Sample hold times were estimated.

A multilinear regression generic model was set up. This model thereby is only applicable for comparable sampling procedures, sampling equipment, offline method and the process conditions used. Sample hold times thereby have a relatively small effect and could be dismissed without altering the general outcome.

Equation (1): generic model to estimate sample-based offline pCO_2 [%] by exhaust carbon dioxide [%], bioreactor pH and sample hold time [minutes]:

$$CO_2(aq) = -53.893 + 1.343 * CO_2 - 0.0461 * (CO_2 - 11.453)^2 + 7.908 * pH + 0.376 * hold\ time \quad (1)$$

3. Results

3.1. Media Specific Correlations of the pH and Corresponding Carbon Dioxide Concentration

Media specific correlations of the two independent production media lots manufactured (10k scale) are shown in Figure 2. Although the difference between individually fitted correlations is significant ($p = 0.00222$), the difference in the resulting pH calculated from each correlation was <0.01. For this respective product, data points from two media lots were fitted together, resulting in residuals <0.02 for each data point from the fit model. Lot-to-lot variability was considered negligible in this case.

Equation (2): quadratic equation to calculate pH with the exhaust carbon dioxide concentration (CO_2, [%]) in equilibrium Media Lot A [%] rounded:

$$pH = 7.329 - 0.0636 * CO_2 + (CO_2 - 5.646) * ((CO_2 - 5.646) * 0.0046) \quad (2)$$

Equation (3): quadratic equation to calculate pH with the exhaust carbon dioxide concentration (CO_2 [%]) in equilibrium Media Lot B [%] rounded:

$$pH = 7.331 - 0.0623 * CO_2 + (CO_2 - 5.765) * ((CO_2 - 5.765) * 0.0045) \tag{3}$$

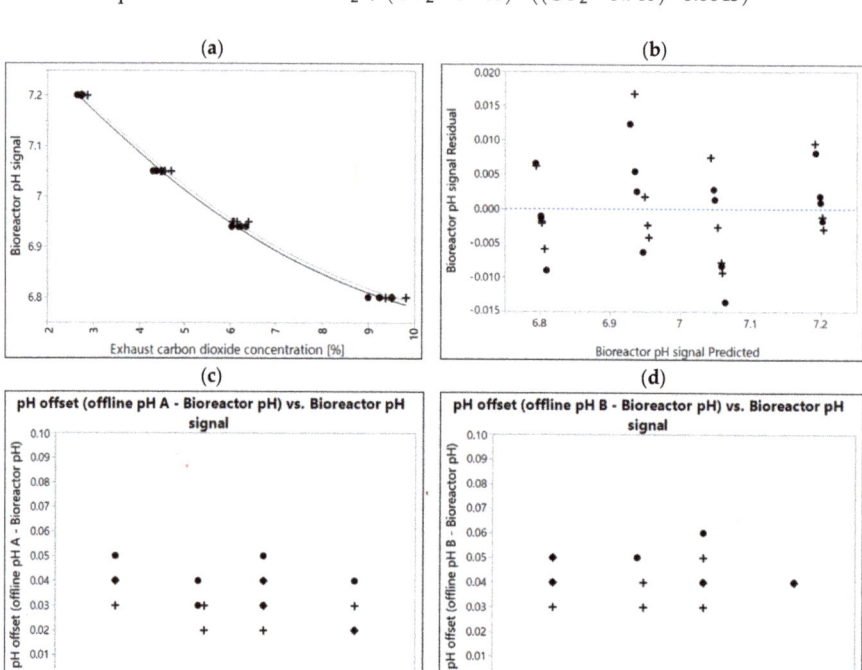

Figure 2. (**a**) A correlation of bioreactor pH and corresponding exhaust carbon dioxide concentration in two different media lots manufactured independently (10k scale). Correlations of lot A (black dots) and lot B (plusses) were experimentally determined in 2 L, N = 4 at different points in time (two weeks apart). The line and dotted line are quadratic fits. Overpressure 300 mbar, Temperature 37 °C. If data of two independent experiments given in (**a**) are fitted together, residuals of combined fit (**b**) still range between ± 0.02 pH. (**c**,**d**) difference sample-based offline value from bioreactor pH ranging between 0.02 and 0.06 determined with two independent pH-meters.

For each data point a sample-based offline pH value has also been determined (Figure 2a,b). Calibration procedure for the pH meters is stricter here than criteria for most products allow. Furthermore, conditions for sampling and sample-based offline measurement are usually more defined in small-scale labs vs. large-scale manufacturing. Therefore, offsets shown here may be considered best case, and highlight the maximum accuracy that can be achieved using sample-based offline measurement in this case. All offsets are positive. This is typical in cell free media and can be explained by temperature (measurements were performed at 32 ± 2 °C compared to 37 °C in the bioreactor) as well as carbon dioxide degassing effects during sampling, sample hold time and measurement. Although pH meters were calibrated in identical buffers and were measuring identical samples, individual data points may already differ by up to 0.03 pH.

Although one single offline value may not represent the true bioreactor pH, it is possible to estimate an average offset to the true pH (Figure 3). This may be especially helpful to determine local offsets that may vary between sites for transfer purposes. The higher the variability of the respective local offsets between sample-based offline measurements and the true pH of the cell environment, the higher the risk of making a GMP decision (like readjusting bioreactor pH-probe signal) that is based on a flawed reading. Averages therefore have to be considered with care, depending on the implemented pH readjustment strategy.

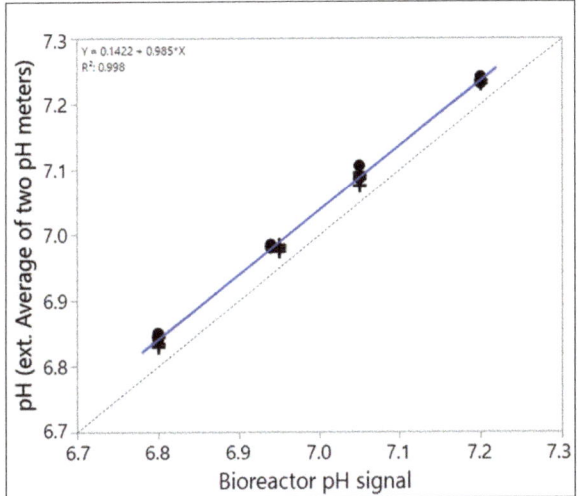

Figure 3. Average of sample-based offline values of two pH-meters compared to the bioreactor pH signal that reflects the true pH in the case shown in Figure 2. Clearly, an offset is detectable that averages around 0.04 pH in this case.

3.2. Effect of pH Correction Agent on Media Specific Correlations of the pH and Corresponding Carbon Dioxide Concentration

Media preparation procedures directly affect correlations like the ones shown in Figure 2a. The most relevant ingredients are solutions at extreme pH or the pH correction agent itself. Dosing and weighing tolerances may add some additional variability as well. The effect of the pH correction agent on the exhaust carbon dioxide concentration at a given pH in consecutive bioreactors where pH is controlled via carbon dioxide gas as the acidic component is shown in Figure 4. In this case, an increase of around 0.5% carbon dioxide in the exhaust would result in a pH difference of around 0.03 pH in this medium given the correlation shown in Figure 2a. If the effect of correction agent is well known, acceptance criteria can be derived to assess if the method is feasible even if media preparation itself introduces some errors. When a certain correlation is used to calculate pH from the exhaust carbon dioxide concentration, varying amounts of pH correction agent that are added during media preparation to counteract, e.g., carbon dioxide removal will add error to the method.

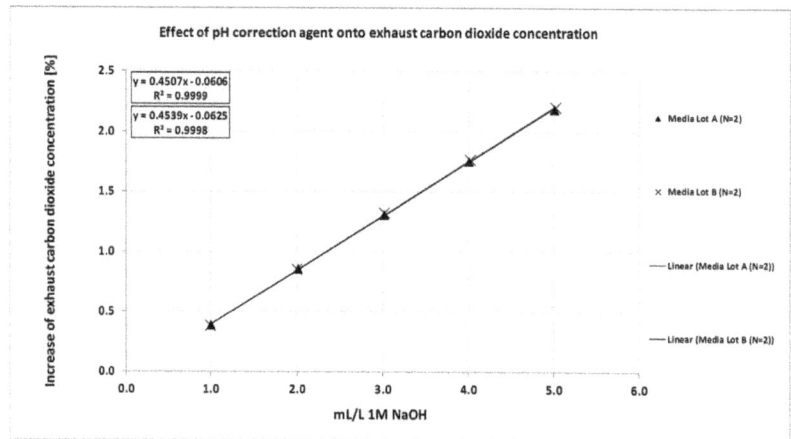

Figure 4. Effect of pH correction agent 1 M NaOH on the exhaust carbon dioxide concentration in 2 L bioreactor systems with active pH control and carbon dioxide gas as the acidic component. In the range tested, the correlation is linear and almost identical between media lots.

3.3. Determination of Offsets between Sample-Based Offline Measurement and Carbon Dioxide Derived pH for Validation

Offsets and distributions of the difference between sample-based offline measurement and the pH derived by a correlation pH and corresponding exhaust carbon dioxide concentration are shown in Figure 5. Data were determined in a GMP manufacturing line for a legacy product with a production scale of 5000 L as part of the validation efforts for this product. Scale independency for this product was shown in 20 L as described in Materials and Methods. Furthermore, equivalence of the offsets between sample-based offline values and bioreactor pH in scales 10 L, 50 L, 500 L and 5000 L were proven with two one sided *t*-tests (TOST) using double the standard deviation of historic differences between online and offline pH values as practically significant differences.

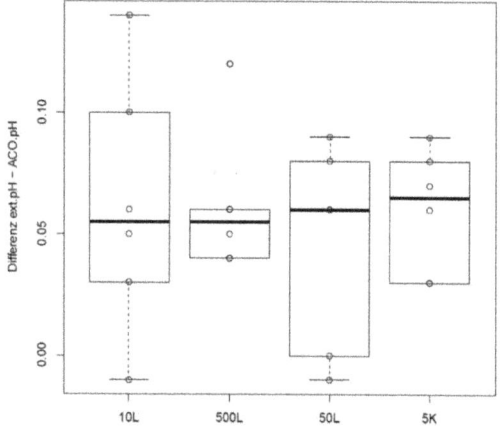

Figure 5. Difference of sample-based offline values and pH calculated from the exhaust carbon dioxide concentration depending on scale.

Offsets introduced by sample-based offline measurements obviously do not differ significantly between scales in this case. It must be noted that even if respective mean difference is within the defined PSDs, offset of a single data point may vary tremendously in reality. Compared to the offset and variability shown for the small scale data in Figures 1 and 2, it becomes clear that sampling and calibration procedures on the manufacturing floor may introduce offsets and variability that affects process performance. If the decision to readjust bioreactor probes is based on one single sample-based offline reading, true pH may already vary by about 0.1 pH, looking at this dataset alone.

3.4. Feasibility of the Carbon Dioxide-Derived pH in Single Use Bioreactors

The time for the equilibration phase depended on vessel size, headspace to working volume ratio and aeration rates and did partially take up to 9 h on a 2K scale.

Scalability and particularly the robustness of this method are shown in Figure 6. pH in all runs in all scales was calculated from a quadratic fit generated on a small scale as described above. Figure 6 compares pH values derived from exhaust carbon dioxide concentration vs. sample-based offline measurement in 250 L SUBs.

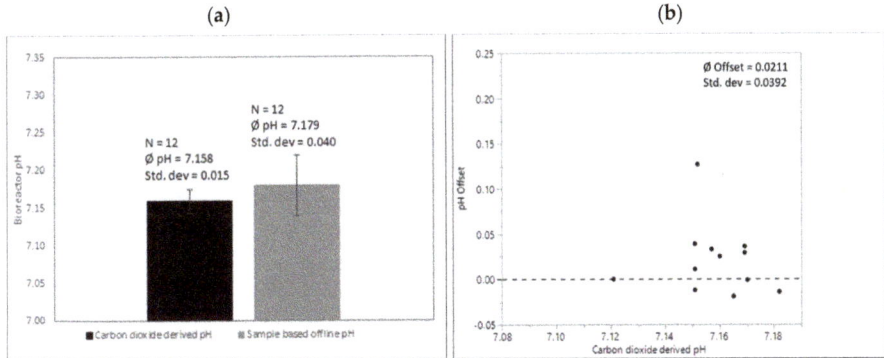

Figure 6. (a) Comparison of carbon dioxide-derived and sample-based pH before inoculation after media fill. pH-probe signals were adjusted onto correlation exhaust carbon dioxide concentration and corresponding pH in all 250 L SUBs. Processes were executed from various operators over a period of several months with the same culture media recipe and the same conditions at the calibration time point as described above. (b) pH offset of sample-based offline values compared to quadratic fit for correlation exhaust carbon dioxide concentration and corresponding pH.

Again, an almost negligible mean difference between the sample-based and carbon dioxide-derived pH can be observed (0.021). However, the standard deviation of the sample-based offline measurement compared to the proposed method again reflects a high variability. This highlights that mean offsets might differ depending on local procedures, but all sample-based offline methods potentially add a high pH variability to cell culture operations. An offset of >0.1 for a single data point is not unusual.

Sample-based offline measurements via automated liquid handling in Ambr250™ systems compared to pH derived by exhaust carbon dioxide concentrations are shown in Figure 7.

As mentioned, sample exposition to a CO_2-free environment has to be considered high, impacting pH via carbon dioxide degassing. Offsets were mainly positive with a mean difference of around 0.05. Again, variability is high adding variability to cell culture operations if single data points are used to adjust respective bioreactor pH-probe signals.

After transferring the quadratic fit formula into clinical GMP manufacturing, carbon dioxide concentrations of two 2k SUBs with more or less comparable media fill and equilibration procedures were determined and the pH was calculated (Figure 8).

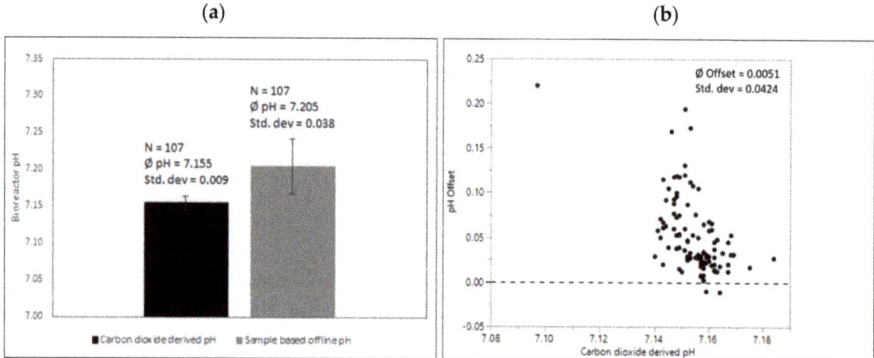

Figure 7. (a) Comparison of carbon dioxide-derived and sample-based pH before inoculation after media fill. Processes were executed from various operators over a period of several months with the same culture media recipe and the same conditions at the calibration time point as described. (b) pH offsets of sample-based offline values compared to quadratic fit for correlation exhaust carbon dioxide concentration and corresponding pH. Due to its small volume and automated handling, exposure to carbon dioxide free environmental conditions is considered high.

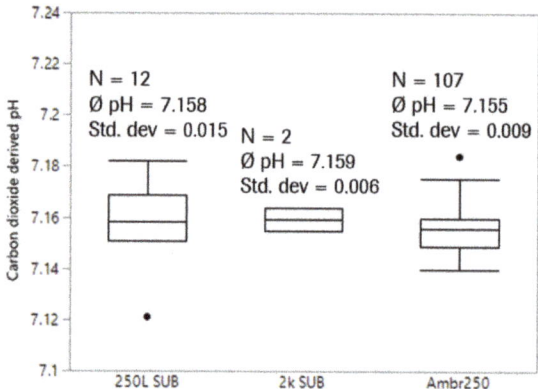

Figure 8. Comparison of carbon dioxide-derived pH after media fill before inoculation between scales and plants. pH offline values for 2k SUBs had an offset of 0.009 and 0.046, respectively.

pH values derived from the exhaust carbon dioxide concentration are obviously very comparable and show low variability. Although many potential sources of error exist including media lot-to-lot differences, environmental pressure changes, slight differences in pressure and temperature control to name a few, knocking out offsets by avoiding sampling and sample-based offline measurement does affect comparability and precision of pH measurement using the proposed method.

3.5. Online pCO_2 Monitoring Potential

Trends of the raw exhaust CO_2 concentration measured by the off-gas analyzer as well as pCO_2 modelled as described above are shown in Figure 9. Sample-based offline pCO_2 measurements using a blood gas analyzer are shown as well. All systems had active pressure and temperature control with identical set points.

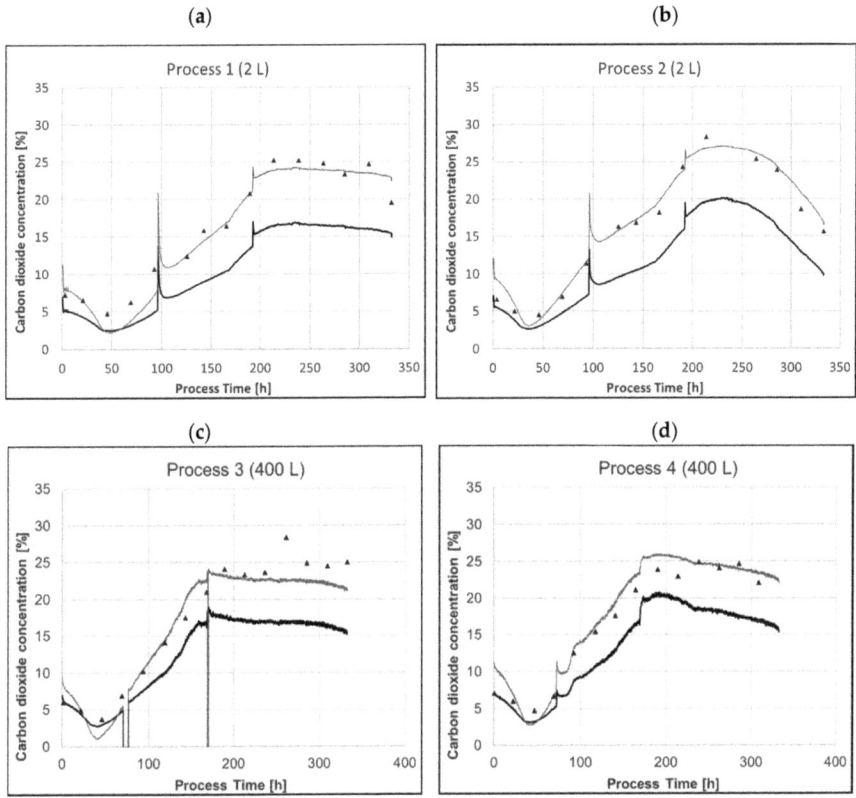

Figure 9. (**a**,**b**) Profiles of raw exhaust CO_2 concentration (black line), predicted pCO_2 concentration using Equation (1) with a sample hold time of 3 min (**a**) or 4.5 min (**b**) (grey line) and the sample-based pCO_2 measurement (black triangles) of a representative process in a 2 L system. (**c**,**d**) Profiles of exhaust CO_2 concentration (black line), of predicted pCO_2 concentration using Equation (1) with a sample hold time of 1 min (grey line) of a representative process in a 400 L system. The model was derived from 2 L data and directly applied to 400 L. All bioreactors were pressure controlled at 400 mbar overpressure.

Exhaust-gas analysis can predict offline pCO_2 relatively accurately with very little effort. Applying the model derived from 2 L data to 400 L runs show the potential for scalability and transferability of those models. Even using the raw carbon dioxide signal represents the trend very well. The main driver for the raw data not directly representing pCO_2 is the applied overpressure. The system pressure directly affects mass transfer from the compressed gas phase to the liquid phase. Analysis of the exhaust gas takes place at environmental pressure. That means that a simple correction to the overall system pressure in the respective bioreactor already provides a more rational way compared to a generic model to correct raw off-gas signal. Events like basic feed additions and resulting pH controller response to counteract pH shifts are perfectly detectable using the raw signal alone. The modelled pCO_2 obviously underestimated the sample-based offline pCO_2 after inoculation. Inoculation and dependent pH controller response lead to immediate changes in dissolved carbon dioxide levels, whereas headspace back mixing takes more time depending on aeration rate. Fast changes like base additions, set point changes or feed additions will have a delayed response in off-gas analysis. Relatively slow process changes in mammalian cell culture processes still allow for meaningful monitoring via exhaust carbon dioxide.

4. Discussion

Sample-based offline measurement of pH and pCO_2 may not represent the true pH in the bioreactor with an accuracy that is required in the future. Many parameters potentially affect sample pH and pCO_2 after sampling. In particular, pH is a parameter that has tremendous impact on process performance. Bioreactor probe signals must be considered a function of respective sample-based offline measurement after readjustment. Procedures to calibrate pH probes that are stated in respective Pharmacopeias or technical references issued by, e.g., the National Institute of Standards and Technology (NIST), are all based on certified pH buffers. Those buffers are designed to be as stable and as independent to environmental conditions like temperature as possible. However, this approach does not necessarily guarantee comparable results in samples that contain cells in cell culture media. Sample properties, sample hold times and local equipment and procedures may alter sample pH in different ways between sites, plants or even operators. Furthermore, buffers are commonly used for sensor calibration at temperatures other than sample temperature, which cannot be compensated for with typical automatic temperature compensation (ATC). Keeping sample temperatures constant is one way to achieve more comparable results. On the other hand reheating cooled samples to fermentation temperature includes longer sample hold times, again altering sample pH. A reference method to prove pH comparable between sites does not yet exist, because samples cannot be measured simultaneously at two sites. Furthermore, samples containing cells cannot be stored or shipped to measure pH somewhere else because effects of cells and the carbonate buffer system would unpredictably alter sample pH.

In this paper, we propose a method that is able to resolve pH with superior accuracy compared to sample-based offline measurement. Because pH can be determined without the need to sample, all potential offsets introduced by sample-based offline measurement are avoidable. Off-gas analysis thereby is relatively easy to establish in GMP manufacturing because measurement takes place outside the sterile barrier. The underlying fundamental chemical principal is very well described and can universally be applied.

The proposed method for pH determination is applicable in cell free media. After inoculation, exhaust carbon dioxide concentration becomes a sum parameter affected mainly by respiration, feed addition, lactate generation and pH controller response. After adjustment of bioreactor pH-probe signals based on the exhaust carbon dioxide concentration, further adjustments based on offline measurement should be avoided. This may question standard pH readjustment strategies based on frequent offline measurement as a detection measure for unintended bioreactor probe drifts.

How well a potential bioreactor probe drift is detectable with offline measurement heavily depends on changing sample properties during fermentation and the overall variability of a respective sample-based offline measurement. Variability directly affects the information content of a single data point derived by, e.g., daily sampling. The data shown alone shows that mean offsets may be small, but overall variability of sample-based offline measurement massively decreases efficacy to accurately determine the true pH in bioreactors.

For internal purposes, delta probe alarms were utilized to detect single probe drifts online in bioreactors that are equipped with more than one pH probe. Probability of an undetectable double probe drift thereby is considered low. Having efficient detectability measures in place to identify potential bioreactor probe drifts thereby reduces the dependency on sample-based offline measurements.

When pH can be determined by exhaust carbon dioxide concentration, pCO_2 can be derived by the very same principles as well. The main advantage is that there is no need for balancing; carbonate concentrations in feed and media solutions as well as carbonate influx simply do not matter for deriving a continuous online signal that is superior to offline values. Data quality derived by pCO_2 probes thereby may be questionable if either are calibrated by defined gas flow added by mass flow controllers or by sample-based offline readings. Accuracy of both methods is limited, leading to limited accuracy of pCO_2 probe signals.

We presented this here together with pH to highlight that having to validate methods against a standard that is flawed by sampling and offline measurement proves difficult. Knowing that offsets are unavoidable for both pH and pCO_2, strong rationales or scientific principles are needed to implement more accurate methods, even if they do not necessarily match the reference due to those offsets. We have to finally accept that a standard that obviously was sufficient for decades may not be sufficient in the future.

For scaling purposes, addressing carbon dioxide removal is extremely easy using off-gas analysis. Carbon dioxide removal equals gas flow times carbon dioxide exhaust concentration. This enables one to directly address aeration strategies without the need to know bioreactor configuration and the usual parameters like $k_L a$, which are notoriously insufficient to match carbon dioxide removal and solubility between a small and large scale.

5. Conclusions

The true bioreactor pH cannot be accurately determined with sample-based offline measurements. Sample-based offline measurements may furthermore be efficient detection measures only for bioreactor pH-probe drifts that are relatively large.

Therefore, we recommend decreasing the dependency on sample-based offline measurements as far as possible. The proposed carbon dioxide-derived method represents a suitable alternative that is applicable in a variety of fermentation systems like stainless steel or single use bioreactors with acceptable effort. In fact, the method described here already has been successfully used for process transfers from a 2 L (Development) up to 12k scale (GMP Manufacturing); not one single sample-based offline pH value has been used to adjust bioreactor probes in the process.

If a sample-based offline measurement is used, we encourage authors to describe exactly how pH was measured including sample hold times, offline methods, calibration routines and readjustment strategies. Findings are not necessarily reproducible if the pH control strategy is unknown, making scientific progress in mammalian cell culture especially slow.

The ability to control pH more accurately will have tremendous impact on many industrial needs in the future. Bringing down process variability finally enables us to detect other effectors that are now undetectable and unquantifiable due to underlying process variability, and this variability is significantly driven by pH variability. The impact of raw materials, seed train and inoculum train operations, media preparation and so on will be better quantifiable.

More sophisticated approaches, such as complex modelling and soft sensoring, proteomics/transcriptomics, in silico approaches, and advanced analytics that also depend on pH, will only yield more relevant findings if data quality increases. Current pH variability in mammalian cell culture inhibits faster progress in all areas related to mammalian cell culture, and the potential of tighter and more accurate pH control cannot be underestimated.

6. Patent Applications

WO/2017/072340 MONITORING STATE DEVIATIONS IN BIOREACTORS, PCT/EP/2016/076167 Applicant F.HOFFMANN-LA ROCHE AG.

WO/2017/072346 IDENTIFICATION OF CALIBRATION DEVIATIONS OF PH-MEASURING DEVICES, PCT/EP/2016/076173 Applicant F.HOFFMANN-LA ROCHE AG.

Author Contributions: Conceptualization C.K., Methodology C.K., formal analysis T.W. for SUBs, V.T. for pCO_2, C.K. for pH reference method writing—original draft preparation, C.K., V.T., T.W. writing—review and editing, C.K., V.T., T.W.; visualization, C.K., V.T., T.W. All authors have read and agreed to the published version of the manuscript.

Funding: This work is exclusively funded by F. Hoffmann-La Roche AG.

Acknowledgments: This work is a small excerpt of a global development and implementation initiative within the Roche Drug Substance Network, where people of all functions including regulatory, procurement, manufacturing, development, research, quality functions and management drive and fund ongoing efforts. Eppendorf and BlueSens were especially supportive providing in-depth knowledge and device upgrades for GMP implementation.

Conflicts of Interest: Author Christian Klinger is also Inventor of the carbon dioxide-based pH reference method and therefore has a potential conflict of interest. F. Hoffmann-La Roche AG is funder and owner of the patent application *"the carbon dioxide based pH reference method"* and therefore has a potential conflict of interest. The funders had no role in the design of the study; in the collection, analyses, or interpretation of data; in the writing of the manuscript, or in the decision to publish the results. Certainly, the funders had particular interest in the outcome and benefits that may be realized by developing and implementing the proposed method.

References

1. Michl, J.; Park, K.C.; Swietach, P. Evidence-based guidelines for controlling pH in mammalian live-cell culture systems. *Commun. Biol. Vol.* **2019**, *2*, 144. [CrossRef] [PubMed]
2. de Pool, J.D.; Van Den Berg, S.A.; Pilgram, G.S.; Ballieux, B.E.; Van Der Westerlaken, L.A. Validation of the blood gas analyzer for pH measurements in IVF culture medium: Prevent suboptimal culture conditions. *PLoS ONE* **2018**, *13*, e0206707. [CrossRef] [PubMed]
3. Frahm, B.; Blank, H.C.; Cornand, P.; Oelssner, W.; Guth, U.; Lane, P.; Munack, A.; Johannsen, K.; Pörtner, R. Determination of dissolved CO(2) concentration and CO(2) production rate of mammalian cell suspension culture based on off-gas measurement. *J. Biotechnol.* **2002**, *99*, 133–148. [CrossRef]
4. Lawrence, J. Henderson. Concerning the relationship between the strength of acids and their capacity to preserve neutrality. *Am. J. Physiol.* **1908**, *21*, 173–179.
5. Busse, C.; Biechele, P.; de Vries, I.; Reardon, K.F.; Solle, D.; Scheper, T. Sensors for disposable bioreactors. *Eng. Life Sci.* **2017**, *17*, 940–952. [CrossRef]

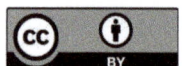

© 2020 by the authors. Licensee MDPI, Basel, Switzerland. This article is an open access article distributed under the terms and conditions of the Creative Commons Attribution (CC BY) license (http://creativecommons.org/licenses/by/4.0/).

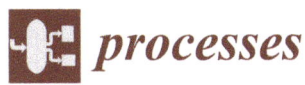

Article

A Reliable Automated Sampling System for On-Line and Real-Time Monitoring of CHO Cultures

Alexandra Hofer [1], Paul Kroll [1,2], Matthias Barmettler [3] and Christoph Herwig [1,2,*]

1. Research Area Biochemical Engineering, Institute of Chemical, Environmental and Biological Engineering, Vienna University of Technology, Gumpendorferstrasse 1a-166/4, 1060 Vienna, Austria; alexandra.hofer@protonmail.com (A.H.); kroll.paul@protonmail.com (P.K.)
2. CD Laboratory on Mechanistic and Physiological Methods for Improved Bioprocesses, Vienna University of Technology, Gumpendorferstrasse 1a-166/4, 1060 Vienna, Austria
3. Securecell AG, In der Luberzen 29, 8902 Urdorf, Switzerland; matthias.barmettler@securecell.ch
* Correspondence: christoph.herwig@tuwien.ac.at; Tel.: +43-1-58801-166400

Received: 30 April 2020; Accepted: 23 May 2020; Published: 27 May 2020

Abstract: Timely monitoring and control of critical process parameters and product attributes are still the basic tasks in bioprocess development. The current trend of automation and digitization in bioprocess technology targets an improvement of these tasks by reducing human error and increasing through-put. The gaps in such automation procedures are still the sampling procedure, sample preparation, sample transfer to analyzers, and the alignment of process and sample data. In this study, an automated sampling system and the respective data management software were evaluated for system performance; applicability with HPLC for measurement of vitamins, product and amino acids; and applicability with a biochemical analyzer. The focus was especially directed towards the adaptation and assessment of an appropriate amino acid method, as these substances are critical in cell culture processes. Application of automated sampling in a CHO fed-batch revealed its potential with regard to data evaluation. The higher sampling frequency compared to manual sampling increases the generated information content, which allows easier interpretation of the metabolism, extraction of e.g., k_s values, application of smoothing algorithms, and more accurate detection of process events. A comparison with sensor technology shows the advantages and disadvantages in terms of measurement errors and measurement frequency.

Keywords: automated sampling; process analytical technology; CHO; bioprocess; amino acids; vitamins

1. Introduction

The performance of even complex bioprocesses depends on their control. Often, the bottleneck is how and if relevant process variables can be monitored. In red biotechnology, for example, complex expression systems such as Chinese hamster ovary (CHO) cells are widely used for the production of biopharmaceuticals. These processes are very sensitive to small variations caused by known and unknown disturbances such as raw material, process, and biological variances. In order to ensure acceptable reliable process performance, powerful monitoring is the key [1]. Regarding mammalian cell culture processes, a variety of substances such as glucose (as the main C-source), amino acids, fatty acids, product (mAb), and metabolites are involved. Each one of them could affect process performance by limiting or inhibiting effects. In addition, the often very low concentration of the analytes may be a challenge or even an exclusion criterion for established monitoring technologies [2]. This results in a huge complexity during process development, scale up, and production. To overcome such limitations, monitoring strategies based on automated sampling seem promising [3]. For the realization of timely measurements, a combination of automated sampling, sample processing, and sample analysis is required [4]. Such a monitoring system must be robust (processing of on-line and off-line samples), accurate, flexible, and easy to use. The acquired data should lead to the possibility for improvement, resulting in an increase of process robustness.

In order to fulfill these requirements, a system for automated sampling as well as the analytical methodology are crucial. Common ways for automated sampling include a membrane immersion nozzle, which is prone to membrane fouling and protein adsorption [5–7]. A reliable system must take a culture broth sample and process it in the reactor environment. This can also facilitate the flexibility of analyzing the culture broth itself or the supernatant. The analytical method chosen should best be the reference method, which is normally bound to the analytical stream and can just be applied off-line. High performance liquid chromatography (HPLC) is a common reference analyzer used for the analysis of substrates, metabolites, and product or product quality attributes. Consequently, it also delivers a high amount of flexibility.

In terms of Process Analytical Technology (PAT), critical process parameters (CPP) must be monitored and controlled [8]. In CHO processes, important parameters for process performance are often amino acids [9–11]. Investigation of the amino acid profile during cultivation is essential to establish an efficient feeding strategy. The limiting amino acids differ from process to process. If assessed at all, state-of-the-art is off-line HPLC analysis using sample derivatization, which is often performed manually. On-line availability of these data would allow faster generation of process understanding to establish feeding and control strategies and finally reduce time-to-market.

With the evaluation of a system for automated sampling and sample processing, we want to close the gap between reference analytics and the process stream to enable process monitoring in terms of PAT. The system was evaluated by a CHO process, applying on-line HPLC and a biochemical analyzer for analysis of substrates, metabolites, and products.

The following four points sum up the investigated challenges of the sample-based monitoring system:

- Quantification of the automated liquid handling and analysis
- Optimization and adaptation of an HPLC method for amino acid measurement
- Application on a mammalian cell culture fed batch
- Comparison to other real-time monitoring systems

2. Materials and Methods

2.1. Chemicals and Reagents

All chemicals and substances were of analytical grade and purchased from either Carl Roth (Karlsruhe, Germany) or Sigma Aldrich (St. Louis, MO, USA). For analytical methods, ultra-pure water was used, derived from a Milli-Q system from Merck Millipore (Billerica, MA, USA).

2.2. HPLC Methods

Vitamins were analyzed according to Hofer et al. [12].

The chromatographic separation as well as the principle for sample derivatization of amino acids were performed as described in Hofer et al. [13]. In order to facilitate automated on-line analysis, a fraction collector autosampler was used. Hence, the derivatization protocol had to be implemented for in-well derivatization by user defined programming (UDP). In order to reach reliable results, some parameters were evaluated as described in Section 3.1.

IgG was analyzed with a protein A cartridge (Applied Biosystems, Bedford, MA, USA) and detected at 210 nm.

2.3. Biochemical Methods

Glucose, lactate, ammonium, IgG and glutamine were analyzed by the biochemical analyzer Cedex® Bio HT (Roche Diagnostics, Mannheim, Germany).

2.4. Set-Up

The set-up consists of a 3.6 L bioreactor (Labfors 5, Infors HT, Bottmingen, Switzerland) equipped with a pH and a pO_2 (Hamilton, Reno, NV, USA) probe, an off-gas sensor (BlueInOne, BlueSens gas sensor GmbH, Herten, Germany), six scales, and three additional peristaltic pumps. One port is occupied by an immersion nozzle, which is directly connected to the multiplexer module (MUX) of the automated sampling system Numera (Securecell AG, Urdorf, Switzerland). The automated sampler is a modular system that was equipped with the MUX, a dilution module (SDU), a filtration module (TFU), a routing module (SRU), a control panel (CPU), and an autosampler (ASX). The implemented SRU allows various combinations of sample processing, i.e., dilution and filtration. The Numera was connected to two analyzers, namely an HPLC and a Cedex® Bio HT (Roche Diagnostics, Mannheim, Germany) (Figure 1). The Ultimate 3000 HPLC (Thermo Fisher Scientific, Waltham, MA, USA) was equipped with a pump (LPG-3400SD), an autosampler (WPS-3000FC), a column compartment (TCC-3000SD), a diode array detector (DAD-3000), and a fluorescence detector (FLD-3400RS). The connection between the Numera and the HPLC depends on the methods applied at the HPLC. For methods that require a simple direct injection of the particle free sample, the tubings of the pump and column compartment are directly connected with the injection valve of the ASX. The HPLC autosampler is not used in that case. If the method requires some preprocessing of the particle free samples, the valve of the ASX is linked with the fraction collector valve of the HPLC autosampler. This way, the sample can be transported into deep well-plates in the HPLC autosampler and sample processing can be performed there in the same way as with off-line samples. The Cedex® Bio HT is connected via a liquid path between the SRU module and a fixed cuvette in one of the sample racks.

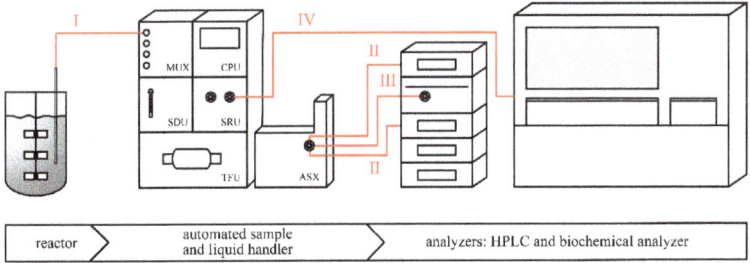

Figure 1. The set-up applied for the experiments consisted of a bioreactor, an automated sampling system (Numera), an HPLC, and a Cedex® Bio HT. The red lines indicate the path of the sample in a very simplified manner. In path I, the sample is drawn from the bioreactor to the sterile barrier of the MUX via an immersion nozzle. According to applied sample processing, the paths in the Numera between the modules can differ, but finally all end in the ASX for sample collection. The injection valve of the ASX can directly connect the HPLC pump and column, hence it can directly inject the sample into the HPLC (path II). If an autosampler is required at the HPLC, both sampler injection valves can be connected and the sample is transferred to the HPLC sampler (path III). A sample for the Cedex® Bio HT is transported from the ASX to the SRU, which is connected with a sample rack of the Bio HT for sampler transfer (path IV).

2.5. The Automated Sampling System

The sterility of the bioprocess was maintained as follows: the immersion nozzle coupled to a sampling line was connected to the bioreactor and sterilized by autoclavation with the bioreactor. After autoclavation, the sampling line is inserted in a pinch valve at the multiplexer module and connected to the module. The pinch valve opens only when the sample is drawn, preventing unsterile liquid to cross the sterile barrier (i.e., the pinch valve). The Numera system supports different sampling procedures. In this study, one sampling procedure was performed and the sample was then transferred to two different analyzers, namely HPLC and Bio HT (Figure 2). The inner diameter of the immersion nozzle of 0.8 mm, the ability of the MUX to backflush excessive sample with sterile air, and the proximity of reactor to Numera ensure minimal sampling volume.

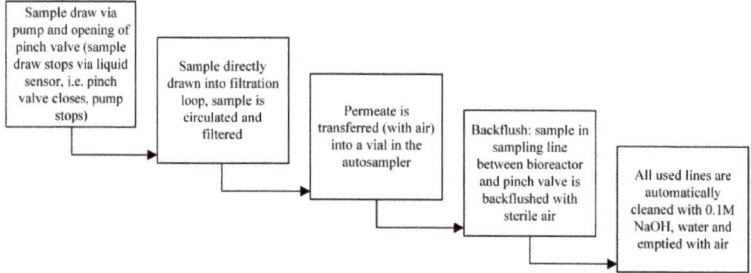

Figure 2. Sampling sequence performed with the system for storage of a cell free sample on the autosampler without dilution. Samples were then transferred via the injection valve on the autosampler to the HPLC or the samples were transferred via a pump on the routing module to the Bio HT.

2.6. Software and Data Management

The combination of three software programs was applied for the set-up: (i) Chromeleon 7.2.7 (Thermo Fisher Scientific, USA) to control the HPLC and to quantify the peak areas (ii) the Cedex® BioHT Analyzer Application Software Version 5.0.0.1206 (Roche Diagnostics, Germany) to control the Bio HT, and (iii) the Process Information Management System Lucullus PIMS (Securecell AG, Switzerland). In order to facilitate the handling of the set-up, the overall control was applied via Lucullus PIMS. All devices attached to the process were connected to Lucullus PIMS, including probes, scales, and pumps as well as the Numera and both analyzers. Hence, automated sampling and sample analysis were triggered via Lucullus PIMS (Figure 3). An analytical trigger initiated the measurements by automatically starting the respective control software for HPLC and Bio HT. Overall, Lucullus was applied for data recording, data sorting and control.

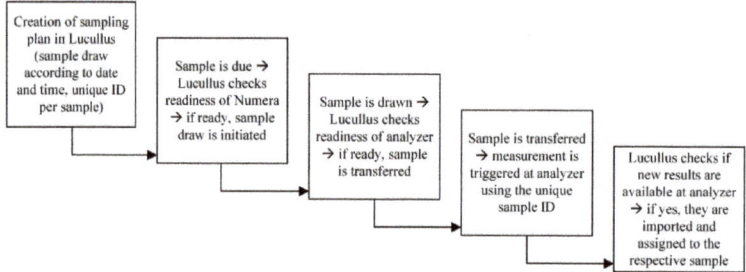

Figure 3. Coordination of the sampling procedure performed by the software Lucullus PIMS.

2.7. Cultivations

CHO cultivations were performed using the set-up described above. The system was supplied with air, O_2, CO_2 and N_2 to control dissolved O_2 at 40.0% and CO_2 at 12.5%, respectively. The pH was controlled at 7.00 with acid and base, and temperature was controlled at 37 °C. In fed-batch mode, three closed-loop feeds were applied. Automated sampling and analysis were applied every 2 or 3 h. Manual sampling was performed every 12 h.

2.8. Technical Run

Sterility was evaluated by a technical bioreactor run after simulation in Matlab® 2017a. The bioreactor was filled with a complex medium and the main process parameters were controlled and set as usual in a CHO process, i.e., pH 7.00, temperature of 37 °C and pO_2 of 40%. After 60 h, a water feed was started, followed by a glucose feed after 120 h. Automated sampling was performed every 6 h and manual sampling every 24 h. The experiment was aborted after 370 h of sterile run time. Sterility was evaluated by microscopic analysis as well as by process parameters such as oxygen inflow.

3. Results

3.1. System Performance

The sample handling of the system was evaluated in experiments without cells testing for system sterility, accuracy, and precision. Microscopic analysis as well as an unchanged pO_2 and oxygen inflow demonstrated sterility over the complete run of 370 h.

The sampling system is equipped with tubings having an inner diameter of 0.75 mm in order to facilitate low sample volumes. Hence, the volume-to-surface ratio is predestined for small liquid residues that might have a high impact on accuracy. This sample dilution was evaluated by comparing on-line and off-line measured samples by HPLC. A distinct sample dilution could be observed when applying the sampling system. Nevertheless, the systematic error can be eliminated by two approaches: (i) calculation of the dilution factor (DF) and inclusion in the sample analysis or (ii) calibration of the analytical device via the Numera system, i.e., the standard solutions are processed via Numera and automatically injected into the HPLC. Both approaches showed high accuracy with a relative deviation from the true value of 0.1% and 3%, respectively (Figure 4A). The differences in the linear correlations between all approaches are listed in Table 1, showing a slope of nearly 1 for both correction methods. It should be noted that the degree of dilution depends both on the number of applied modules and the applied analyzer. With the application of a 1:1 dilution to the drawn sample, the dilution module produces the highest unwanted DF. For dilutions between 1:2 and 1:25, the DF can be reduced to <1% by being integrated into the qualification of the module. Finally, the precision of the system was evaluated. Therefore, a glucose standard was repeatedly sampled, processed, and analyzed with the Cedex® Bio HT. The results show a high precision and reproducibility of the measurement with a bias of 0.31% and relative deviation of 1.1%. The relative deviation is a combination of the deviation caused by the Numera and the Bio HT analyzer (Figure 4B).

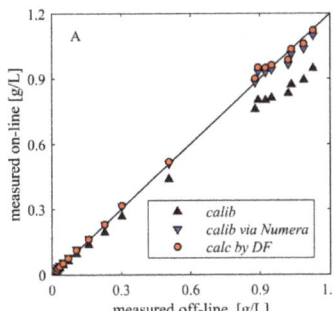
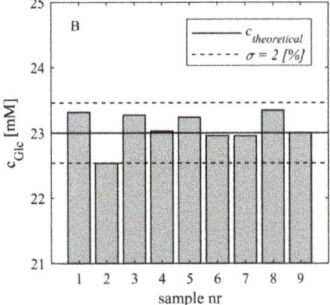

Figure 4. The automated sampling system was assessed for accuracy and precision. (Plot **A**) shows a high accuracy if the systematic error of the occurring sample dilution is considered. This can be achieved by calculating the actual value with a dilution factor or by calibrating the analytical device via the automated sampler. (Plot **B**) illustrates the precision of the measurement after processing the sample with the Numera system with a relative standard deviation of 1%. Additionally, all measurements are located within a 2% interval around the true value.

Table 1. Parameters of the correlations between off-line and on-line measured samples, (i) applying common calibration of the HPLC, (ii) processing calibration standards via Numera or (iii) adjusting the analytical result by multiplying with the calculated DF.

Correlation	Slope	Offset	Confidence Interval Slope (95%)	R2
Off-line vs on-line	0.8409	0.0056	0.8216–0.8602	0.9981
Off-line vs on-line calibrated via Numera	0.9696	0.0133	0.9474–0.9918	0.9981
Off-line vs on-line considering DF	0.9973	0.0067	0.9745–1.0202	0.9981

3.2. Monitoring—HPLC Autosampler Required

Amino acids play an important role in various bioprocesses, especially in CHO cultivations [9–11]. Thus, the monitoring of amino acids might be crucial for process performance. Analysis via HPLC methods require a derivatization step, which can be performed manually, or by automatization via in-needle or in-vial derivatization. In order to facilitate on-line amino acid measurements with the Numera system, an HPLC autosampler (WPS-3000FC, Thermo Fisher Scientific) was included in the set-up. Additionally, an in-needle derivatization method was assessed regarding its feasibility with the system.

First, basic steps within the derivatization method were assessed. Different approaches for the partial loop filling were programmed and tested for highest reproducibility. The method drawing 10 µL water and 30 µL sample resulted in a relative deviation of 0.09%, which was assessed by a twelvefold measurement. The needle of the applied autosampler was split in a capillary and a needle puncturer. This set-up is prone to drops that stick to the capillary and affect the accuracy of the dilutions. Hence, a Design of Experiment (DoE) was performed to evaluate the best washing procedure for the in-vial derivatization. As every additional step increases measurement time and therefore reduces the possible on-line measurement frequency, a compromise between washing and time must be made. The DoE was performed using acetate as test substances to assess the washing procedure of the derivatization method. The factors in the DoE were needle wash, dipping needle in two water vials, and air draw before drawing the next reagent. A fractional factorial design with two levels (on/off) was chosen, resulting in eight experiments and three center points. Every experiment was run in threefold with a water sample after each injection. The responses were (i) precision (i.e., relative standard deviation of each experiment), (ii) carry-over (i.e., average concentration of substance in water sample), and (iii) accuracy (i.e., average offset between measured value and known concentration). The evaluation of the DoE showed that the air draw and an interaction term of needle wash and air draw correlated negatively with precision (Figure 5a). This means that the relative standard deviation is smaller when an air draw or air draw and needle wash were performed. The effect on carry-over showed no significant correlations between any factor and the carry-over. The mean carry-over of all experiments was 0.0040 +/− 0.0049 g/L, which is under the limit of quantification (LOQ) of the analytical method. The evaluation of accuracy resulted in one significant coefficient, the needle wash (Figure 5b). Air draw and two water vial wash showed no significant correlation. As a result, the wash procedure of the derivatization method includes the needle wash as well as the air draw. An additional washing procedure in two water vials was excluded from the final method.

The final derivatization method was assessed by using a method for organic acids. Lactate, acetate, and succinate were pipetted together and diluted with water, mimicking the steps of the derivatization step. Special attention was paid to the step adding the internal standard. Usually, this is performed manually before the automated derivatization starts in the autosampler. In our case, the part had to be included in the derivatization step chain as no manual interference was applied. Reproducibility of the derivatization was evaluated, resulting in a deviation of approx. 2.8% for lactate, acetate, and succinate.

For the final derivatization method, the deviations of the different amino acids were accessed, ranging between 1.35% and 2.68%. Finally, the deviation resulting from the automated sampling system Numera without the method error was determined as 4.5% (Figure 6).

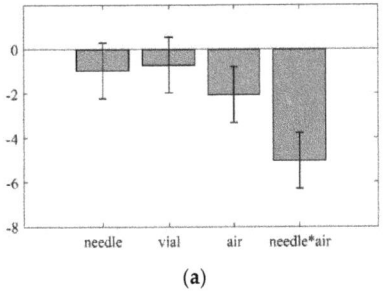 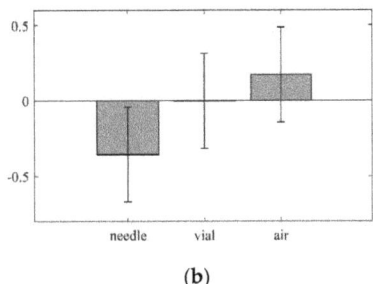

(a) (b)

Figure 5. The coefficient plot (**a**) of the Partial Least Squares (PLS) regression shows the correlation of the different washing procedures on the precision of the derivatization method. The air draw before addition of the next reagent as well as an interaction term of needle wash and air draw show a negative correlation, i.e., these washing procedures result in a higher precision of the method. The underlying model has an R^2 of 0.962 and a Q^2 of 0.477. The coefficient plot (**b**) shows the correlation with the method accuracy. Only needle wash shows a significant negative correlation, i.e., a positive impact on accuracy. The underlying model has an R^2 of 0.590 and a Q^2 of −0.200.

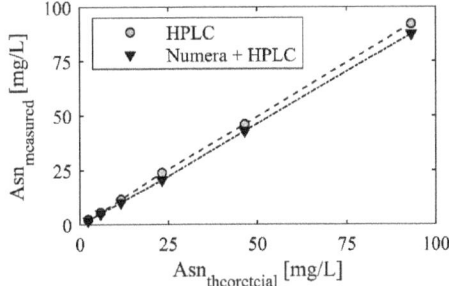

Figure 6. Evaluation of the error of the automated sampling system taking into account the sample draw, filtration, and transfer to the HPLC autosampler. Six standard concentrations of asparagine were analyzed with the developed amino acid derivatization method. The samples were once transferred to the HPLC via Numera (black upside-down triangles) and once injected directly from the HPLC autosampler (grey circles). Comparing the slopes, we receive an error of 4.5% resulting from the transfer and filtration (HPLC slope = 0.9926; Numera + HPLC slope = 0.9475).

In order to be able to transfer the sample via the Numera automated sampling system from the bioreactor to the HPLC autosampler, an HPLC fraction collector autosampler (WPS-3000FC) was used. The injection valve of the autosampler belonging to the Numera automated sampling system was connected with the second injection valve of the WPS-3000FC autosampler of the HPLC, which is normally dedicated to collect fractions after the chromatographic separation. The transfer was performed with a time parameter defining the amount of transferred sample. Along with the transfer, a new injection in the current sequence in Chromeleon was created by the overarching software Lucullus PIMS, coordinating the devices. The instrument method started mixing the sample with the internal standard, followed by the rest of the derivatization procedure and final injection on the column.

Another critical point in the automatization of this analysis is the specific sample dilution needed in order to be within the measurement range of the method. In the beginning, a dilution of 1:50 is required, which exceeds the capabilities of the SDU of the automated sampling system (declared as maximum 1:25 in order to keep a 2% error). Accordingly, for each dilution, a new instrument method was created, applying a dilution step in the beginning of the derivatization procedure and taking into account adjusted amounts of needed internal standard. During the cultivation, the applied instrument method was changed via Lucullus PIMS.

Finally, the method was applied in a CHO process delivering information about the current concentration of 18 different amino acids with a time delay of 45 min after the automated sample draw. Samples were drawn and measured every 3 h. Figure 7 shows the time courses of asparagine (Asn), glycine (Gly), and tyrosine (Tyr) exemplary. For asparagine, the typical sample frequency of once per day and the high frequency of 8 per day are displayed. From a purely visual point of view, it can already be proven at this point that a concentration curve typical of bioprocesses is achieved by a high measuring frequency (second-order kinetic). This cannot be derived from a low-frequency measurement. The reason for this is the information content, which can be explained by the fisher information matrix (1). The parameter n_{SP} represents the number of sampling points. From this follows the simple conclusion that the information about a system increases with the number of observations.

$$H_\theta(\theta,\varphi) = H_\theta^0 + \sum_{k=1}^{n_{sp}} \sum_{i=1}^{N_y} \sum_{j=1}^{N_y} s_{ij} \left[\frac{\partial \hat{y}_i(t_k)}{\partial \theta_l}^T \frac{\partial \hat{y}_j(t_k)}{\partial \theta_m} \right]_{l,m=1...N_\theta} \qquad (1)$$

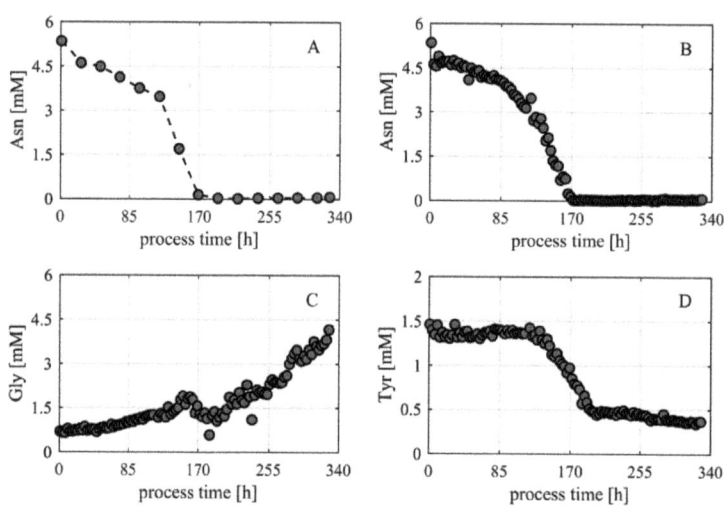

Figure 7. Examples of amino acid concentrations monitored in an automated manner during a CHO cultivation. Plot (**A**) shows the asparagine concentrations received when sampled once per day; plot (**B**) when sampled 8 times per day. High-frequency sampling allows better interpretation of the underlying uptake kinetics. Plot (**C**) shows glycine over time and plot (**D**) tyrosine over time, which was fed.

Not only does this allow more precise statements about the reaction kinetics, but also about the extraction of any process-critical parameters such as k_S values or, with regard to process control, the more accurate detection of process events.

In the process examined, tyrosine was sublimed in an additional feed. The success of the addition can be seen in Figure 7D. The concentration of tyrosine remains almost constant at a level of 0.5 mM (~90 mg/L). Monitoring in this concentration range in a complex mixture of substances is currently not possible with any other on-line technology. As an example, it can be compared with the monitoring of four amino acids with an in-line Raman sensor, which showed a root mean square error of estimation (RMSEE) of the calibration model of 0.41 mM for tyrosine, 0.24 mM for tryptophan, 0.35 mM for phenylalanine, and 0.27 mM for methionine [14]. Unfortunately, the publication shows no concentration of the amino acids over process time.

3.3. Monitoring—HPLC Direct Transfer

HPLC is often applied as reference analytic for product or metabolite analysis. Hence, on-line availability could have a huge impact on process control and time-to-market. If standard HPLC methods are applied that need no addition of internal standard or any other steps such as derivatization, a direct transfer of the sample to the analyzer can be performed. This means that the pump of the HPLC as well as the column are directly connected to the injection valve of the Numera autosampler. The injection is triggered via Lucullus PIMS, the syringe of the Numera autosampler is transferring the sample in the sample loop, and the injection is initiated. Thereby, a full-loop injection is performed, which requires approximately 350 µL of sample to ensure complete filling of the 50 µL sample loop.

The system was applied to generate on-line data of product (IgG) in a fed-batch experiment (Figure A1) and of vitamins in a batch experiment (Figure A2). The product measurement had a runtime of 3 min resulting in a possible sampling frequency of once every 15 min (i.e., time for sample drawing, sample processing, sample injection, and completed HPLC analysis). The vitamin measurement runtime was 26 min, including column washing, resulting in a possible sampling frequency of once every 30 min (sampling and sample processing can be performed while HPLC is still running).

The reliability of the system could be demonstrated in the product analysis. No manual sampling was applied for 50 h during the experiment, relying on automated sampling and on-line analysis.

The possible advantage of high frequency sampling could be shown with the vitamin data. In total, four different B-vitamins could be detected, namely niacinamide, folic acid, B12, and riboflavin. They were available in very low concentrations, complicating the physiological interpretation over process time. For niacinamide, folic acid, and riboflavin, the high frequent on-line data indicated a clear uptake of the substances by the cells, whereas the interpretation of the manual off-line samples is ambiguous. The high data frequency of the on-line samples allows the application of smoothing algorithms without a bias of the result, which eases the calculation of physiological rates.

3.4. Monitoring—Bio HT Direct Transfer

The connection between the sampling system and the Bio HT was realized by a cuvette that was located in a fixed position in one rack of the Bio HT reserved for automated samples. The cuvette has dimensions of 16 × 10 mm. Taking the needle height into account, this results in a minimal volume of 200 µL necessary for several measurements, which is twice the volume compared to a regular measurement using a 1.5 mL reagent tube. In addition, the settings of the Bio HT had to be adapted to allow around the clock analysis, i.e., the begin of day action starts at 01:00 a.m., standby mode and sleep mode were initialized after 60 min each (which is the maximum that can be set). Hence, analysis of the automated samples had to be performed every 2 h as the system is not reachable by Lucullus PIMS when in sleep mode.

Our goal was to achieve a reliable automated measurement of important parameters and at the same time to take as little volume as possible from the bioreactor. Therefore, 3 mL culture broth was taken, resulting in 1.2 mL filtered sample in vials stored in the autosampler of the Numera. It was noted that the filtration settings deliver different volumes, depending on the cell density of the culture broth. A correlation between the so-called Push Out Time (POT) of the filter and the final volume in the vial could be observed. The dependency of viable cell count (VCC) of CHO cells and required POT to achieve a sample volume of 1.2 mL was assessed experimentally. A linear correlation was obtained, which allows to adapt the POT during the process in a reasonable manner (Figure 8). This way it can be guaranteed that enough sample is available for the Bio HT measurement over the whole process. The adaptation of the POT was applied manually but could be automated either by realizing on-line availability of VCC data or by a model estimating the actual VCC.

The Bio HT does not necessarily need particle free samples for analysis. Hence, another solution could be the direct transfer of cell suspension to the Bio HT by the automated sampling system without the inclusion of a filtration step.

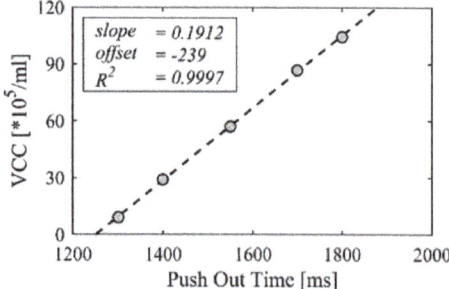

Figure 8. The required POT of the Numera filtration in dependency of the VCC in order to obtain 1.2 mL filtered culture supernatant was assessed experimentally. The linear relationship allows adaptation of the POT during the process to keep the received sample volume constant.

On-line Bio HT analysis was finally applied in a CHO batch process, monitoring glucose, lactate, ammonium, and IgG at a 2 h interval (glucose and lactate shown in Figure 9A). To show the limits of the system on-line analysis was performed every 30 min over 24 h (Figure 9B). As no status feedback of the Bio HT can be sent to Lucullus PIMS by the applied software version of the Bio HT, the 30-min interval is the minimum sampling frequency possible to receive reliable results. A further reduction of the interval could result in a washing of the Bio HT cuvette before the measurement is over and finally in a Bio HT error, interrupting the automated analysis. For the applied sampling intervals, the combination of Numera and Bio HT delivered reliable and precise results, demonstrating its applicability for process monitoring. The variability of the data is linked to measurement error. High concentrations of glucose, which are diluted by the Bio HT, show a greater variance than lactate or glutamine measurements. Nevertheless, the accuracy is high enough to facilitate control actions based on the measurements, especially because control often requires the lower concentration range of glucose.

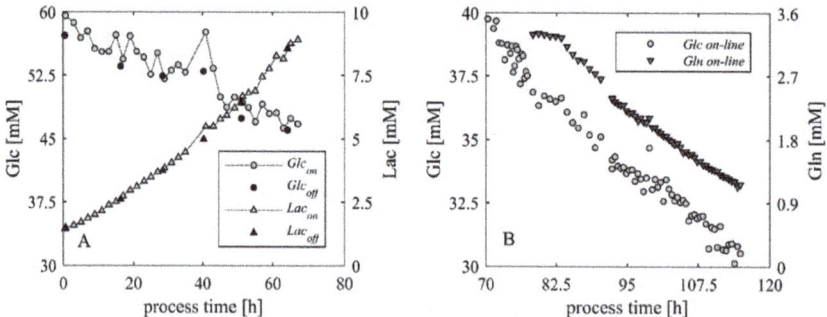

Figure 9. On-line monitoring of substrates and metabolite in a CHO batch process. Plot (**A**) shows the time course of glucose and lactate in the first 70 h of the process with a sampling interval of 2 h. Plot (**B**) shows glucose and glutamine reducing the sampling interval to the minimum of 30 min for 24 h (between 92 h and 116 h of process time).

4. Discussion

4.1. Automated Sampling in General

There are a few scientific contributions available dealing with automated sampling for on-line HPLC [5,6,15–18]. Most of them apply in-situ membrane probes to receive a particle free sample that can be directly injected into an HPLC. The major advantage of these membrane probes is that the membrane is also the sterility barrier. In comparison, the applied system uses a pinch valve in the multiplexer module as sterility barrier, which is in general more prone to failure than a 0.22 µm membrane. On the other hand, a huge disadvantage of the in-situ membrane probes is the membrane fouling that occurs during cultivation as well as the adsorption of proteins, which affects analytical results. A comparison of different membrane probes tackling these challenges was performed by Spadiut et al. [7].

The applied system Numera does not only draw samples but also acts as a liquid handling system. A comparable system, the BaychroMAT®, was presented by Chong et al. [3]. For the BaychroMAT® too, manual and automated samples were compared for glucose, lactate, and viable cell density, resulting in errors between 8.2–14.4%. However, the errors are either higher or comparable to the Numera system.

When applying an automated sampling system, there are a few important points that need to be considered, which were assessed for the commercial automated sampling system Numera:

(1) Does the system impact the sterility of the bioprocess?—No.
(2) How much volume and how much dead volume are drawn from the bioreactor?—The sample volume is approx. 3.5 mL, of which about 1 mL is dead volume.
(3) Does the system support sample processing (i.e., dilution, cell removal etc.)?—Yes.
(4) Does the automated procedure impact the analytical result (i.e., dilution effects)?—There is a constant dilution factor observable, which can be included in final calculations.
(5) How is the communication between process, sampling system, and analyzers realized?—The communication was achieved with one software (Lucullus PIMS) that coordinated the sample draw as well as the transfer of the sample to the analyzer and the initiation of the measurement.

4.2. Assessment of the Presented Liquid Handling System

In summary, the liquid handling system Numera performed very satisfyingly for the required task. The filtration module for cell removal follows an approach using a tape filtration technology and shows some advantages over in-situ filtration probes. However, there are three main aspects that need to be mentioned:

(1) The system was tested for CHO cells with a maximum viable cell density of about $12 \cdot 10^6$ cells/mL, resulting in a required adaptation of the POT to reach the desired volume of permeate after filtration. Currently, the trend is towards high cell density cultivations in perfusion mode, which were not tested in this contribution. The actual filter area in the filtration module is 3.14 cm^2, which is filtering 2.5 mL of cell suspension. An increase of the filter area might have a positive impact on the permeate volume.
(2) During the operation of the system (especially when applying the Protein A HPLC method), it was observed that the precolumn had to be changed approximately 8–10 times during one cultivation run. The required changing frequency increased with progress of the process. This leads to the conclusion that the load of particles of the samples after the automated filtration is higher than after manual cell removal. A reason could be the filtration procedure per se or the applied pore size of the filter of 0.45 µm. Possible solutions to overcome this problem are (i) the use of a membrane with 0.22 µm pore size or (ii) the introduction of a prefiltration step or a dual filtration.

(3) 1–2% of the samples resulted in empty vials after the filtration step.

Another issue that needs further discussion is software communication. In this work, the communication was performed by the software Lucullus PIMS, which coordinated the sample draw via Numera, the transfer to the analyzer, the initiation of the measurement, and the feedback of the analytical results to the other process data. The complexity of the experimental setup used is relatively high, caused by the large number of devices. This requires intensive and frequent support. Common errors were communication problems between the devices. Furthermore, an update of the software of one of the involved devices can lead to communication failure and consequently, system failure. This means that intensive care is needed for the whole setup to guarantee its functionality.

4.3. Comparison with In-Line Sensors

The recent trend for monitoring strategies of substrates and metabolites is towards in-line sensors, especially focusing on spectroscopic methods like Raman [1,2,18,19]. In general, these sensors have some obvious advantages over sample-based monitoring: (i) the methods are non-invasive, (ii) the data frequency is much higher, (iii) the current values of the analytes are available faster, and (iv) the probes have a smaller footprint than for example the described set-up of this contribution. However, there are also some disadvantages that must be considered: (i) in order to interpret spectral data, multivariate tools are needed (e.g., PLS regression models), which require a significant amount of data for model calibration [20]. Hence, a lot of experiments have to be performed that still require manual sampling as well as sample analysis with the respective reference method (e.g., HPLC). (ii) If the calibration model is generated, a continuous validation of the model is necessary, as process disturbances like little variations in the raw material or media may impact the measurement background and with it the calibration model.

In 2018, a contribution was published using Raman spectroscopy for monitoring of four amino acids in a cell culture process [14]. This allows direct comparison of the method using the presented sample-based on-line HPLC approach. First, it should be noted that the sample-based HPLC approach allows monitoring of 18 amino acids in parallel using an established and frequently used methodology, whereas the Raman approach was designed to monitor four amino acids of interest only. Amino acids are typically occurring in the culture supernatant in low concentration (mM range). Comparing the errors of the different methods, it can be shown that the automated HPLC approach leads to an increase in the error by a factor of 3.5 compared to the error of the reference method only, whereas the Raman measurement increased the error 20-fold (Table 2).

Table 2. Comparison of the cv (root mean square error (RMSE)) for four amino acids, with regard to the standard HPLC reference method, the automated sampling with on-line HPLC, and Raman spectroscopy [14].

	Reference Method (HPLC)	Automated Sampling and On-Line HPLC	Raman Spectroscopy
	cv(RMSE) [-]	cv(RMSE) [-]	cv(RMSE) [-]
Tyrosine	0.012	0.058	0.53 *
Tryptophan	0.020	0.066	0.27 *
Phenylalanine	0.016	0.062	0.47 *
Methionine	0.025	0.071	0.29 *

* cv(RMSE) taken from [14].

With regard to an application of the monitoring method for control purposes, not only the error but also the measurement frequency is decisive. The chosen frequency for the Raman measurements was once every 12.5 min (one measurement consisting of 75 scans with an exposure of 10 s per scan) [14]. In comparison, the automated sample-based HPLC method requires approximately 45 min from the beginning of the sample draw till the availability of the analytical result in the process management software. It should be noted that the described sampling system is capable of multiplexing, i.e., up to 16 bioreactors can be connected and sampling procedure is then performed subsequently.

Assuming that 16 bioreactors are connected and only sampled to monitor the amino acids by HPLC as described, this decreases the sampling frequency to once every 12 h.

The authors believe that both methods are highly valuable monitoring tools with different fields of application. Raman spectroscopy is well suited for monitoring manufacturing processes that are designed to be congruent without deviations. The automated sampling approach delivers the opportunity to create more process understanding by applying various methods and is therefore better suited for process development. Furthermore, we believe that a combination of both e.g., by automation of the validation and recalibration of the Raman calibration models could finally be very beneficial.

4.4. Outlook

This contribution focuses on the application of analytical methods with the automated sampling system Numera rather than on the evaluation of the effect of the automated dilution and filtration on cell integrity. A short evaluation has been performed, suggesting that the dilution procedure has no impact on cell viability and the amount of cell debris (Table A1). However, a detailed analysis focusing on e.g., lactate dehydrogenase (LDH) as marker substance for cell integrity should be performed for both preprocessing steps in a further study. Especially, if LDH is a critical process parameter, it must be assured that the automated sampling system has no impact on the analytical result.

Although the application of the sampling system allowed to measure substrates, metabolites, and product in an automated manner, manual samples were still needed to monitor and control the process: (i) Manual samples were needed for the analysis of the viable cell density by a cell counter (Cedex® HiRes, Roche Diagnostics, Germany). The cell count was further used for correlation with a permittivity signal, which was involved in the calculation and control of the feed rates. (ii) Directly after the manual sample draw, pH was measured to check if the calibration of the in-line pH probe requires adjustment.

With regard to product quality, both analyses are essential for nearly every cultivation with mammalian cells [21–26]. Hence, for complete automation of the sampling procedure without any need for additional manual sampling, the analyses of cell count and pH must be automated. In terms of pH measurement, the recalibration procedure of the in-line pH sensor must be automated as well.

5. Conclusions

An advanced PAT set-up was built up including an automated sampling and sample processing system (Numera) enabling HPLC and Cedex® Bio HT as on-line analyzers and applied for CHO cultivations. With regard to the investigated challenges of the sample-based monitoring system, the following conclusions were taken:

- Depending on the preprocessing and the applied analytical method, systematic deviations were observed. They were mainly caused by dilution effects and can be assumed to be constant. On the other hand, the random error seems to be significantly reduced.
- An existing HPLC method for amino acid analysis was successfully adapted in a way that it can now be applied for full automated on-line monitoring.
- The automated sampling and analytic system was successfully tested in mammalian cell culture fed-batch processes. The monitoring of various analytes was performed without significant errors or system failures. The higher measurement frequency and strongly reduced random errors resulted in a larger information content per experiment.
- The accuracy of the system is an order of magnitude better than the compared methods.

Author Contributions: Funding acquisition, C.H.; Investigation, A.H. and P.K.; Methodology, A.H. and M.B.; Resources, C.H.; Supervision, C.H.; Visualization, A.H.; Writing—original draft, A.H. and P.K.; Writing—review & editing, P.K., M.B. and C.H. All authors have read and agreed to the published version of the manuscript.

Funding: This research was funded by Christian Doppler Forschungsgesellschaft, Grant/Award-Number: 171.

Acknowledgments: The authors would like to thank Securecell AG for providing the automated sampling system Numera and the Process Information Management System Lucullus PIMS and Kathrin Oberhuber for English proof reading. The authors acknowledge TU Wien Bibliothek for financial support through its Open Access Funding Program.

Conflicts of Interest: The authors declare no conflict of interest. The funders had no role in the design of the study; in the collection, analyses, or interpretation of data; in the writing of the manuscript, or in the decision to publish the results.

Appendix A

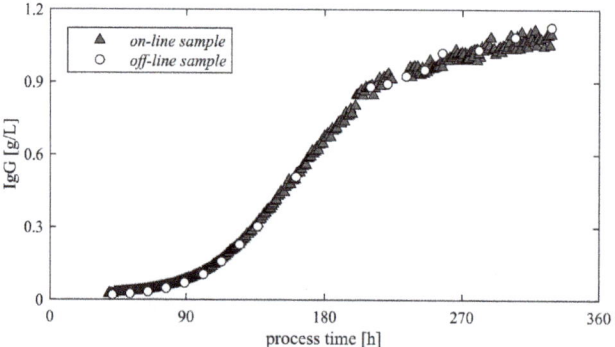

Figure A1. Concentration of product (IgG) in a CHO fed-batch over process time. The grey triangles represent measurements that were performed by the automated sampling and liquid handling system and an on-line HPLC. This data was available in real-time in process management software. The white circles display the corresponding results of the manual samples. Calibration of the HPLC was performed via the Numera system, as described in Section 3.1.

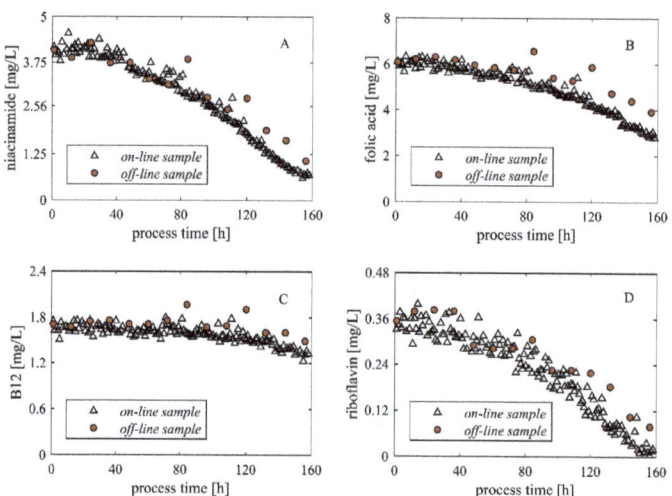

Figure A2. Vitamins were monitored on-line via HPLC. The plots display the concentrations over process time of four different vitamins, i.e., niacinamide in plot A, folic acid in plot B, B12 in plot C and riboflavin in plot D. On-line results (white triangles) and analytical results of manual samples measured off-line (red circles) are compared in each plot. The concentration ranges are very low; hence, high frequency on-line results support interpretation of metabolic behavior of the cells with regard to the analytes.

Table A1. The automated sampling system Numera, especially the dilution module, was roughly evaluated for its impact on cell integrity. CHO cells cultivated in shake flasks were directly analyzed with a cell counter (Cedex® HiRes, Roche Diagnostics, Germany) 5-fold. The same cell suspension was then processed with the Numera system, i.e., drawn from the shake flask, transferred via multiplexer and dilution module, and manually captured after the dilution step. Subsequently, the samples were analyzed with the cell counter. The procedure with Numera was performed two times and each captured sample was analyzed in duplicate. The sample was analyzed for viable cell count (VCC), total cell count (TCC), viability, and cell debris. The results showed no noticeable impact of the Numera system on cell integrity.

Sample	VCC [10^6 Cells/mL]	TCC [10^6 Cells/mL]	Viability [%]	Debris * [10^6 Cells/mL]
Manual 1	3.34	3.44	97.00	0.35
Manual 2	3.45	3.69	93.00	0.48
Manual 3	3.25	3.51	92.70	0.37
Manual 4	3.40	3.62	94.00	0.42
Manual 5	2.79	3.01	92.60	0.48
Numera 1.1	3.68	3.91	94.00	0.47
Numera 1.2	3.29	3.50	94.10	0.57
Numera 2.1	3.27	3.55	92.30	0.43
Numera 2.2	3.14	3.32	94.50	0.45

* debris is defined as cells/particles <7 µm.

References

1. Sonnleitner, B. Automated Measurement and Monitoring of Bioprocesses: Key Elements of the M 3 C Strategy. In *Measurement, Monitoring, Modelling and Control of Bioprocesses*; Springer: Berlin/Heidelberg, Germany, 2012; pp. 1–33.
2. Claßen, J.; Aupert, F.; Reardon, K.F.; Solle, D.; Scheper, T. Spectroscopic sensors for in-line bioprocess monitoring in research and pharmaceutical industrial application. *Anal. Bioanal. Chem.* **2017**, *409*, 651–666. [CrossRef] [PubMed]
3. Chong, L.; Saghafi, M.; Knappe, C.; Steigmiller, S.; Matanguihan, C.; Goudar, C.T. Robust on-line sampling and analysis during long-term perfusion cultivation of mammalian cells. *J. Biotechnol.* **2013**, *165*, 133–137. [CrossRef] [PubMed]
4. Kroll, P.; Sagmeister, P.; Reichelt, W.; Neutsch, L.; Klein, T.; Herwig, C. Ex situ online monitoring: Application, challenges and opportunities for biopharmaceuticals processes. *Pharm. Bioprocess.* **2014**, *2*, 285–300. [CrossRef]
5. Cimander, C.; Bachinger, T.; Mandenius, C.-F. Integration of distributed multi-analyzer monitoring and control in bioprocessing based on a real-time expert system. *J. Biotechnol.* **2003**, *103*, 237–248. [CrossRef]
6. Foley, D.A.; Wang, J.; Maranzano, B.; Zell, M.T.; Marquez, B.L.; Xiang, Y.; Reid, G.L. Online NMR and HPLC as a reaction monitoring platform for pharmaceutical process development. *Anal. Chem.* **2013**, *85*, 8928–8932. [CrossRef]
7. Spadiut, O.; Dietzsch, C.; Posch, A.; Herwig, C. Evaluating online sampling probes for substrate concentration and protein production by a Design of Experiments screening approach. *Eng. Life Sci.* **2012**, *12*, 507–513. [CrossRef]
8. US FDA. Guidance for industry PAT-A Framework for Innovative Pharmaceutical Development, Manufacturing, and Quality Assurance. Available online: www.fda.gov/downloads/Drugs/Guidances/ucm070305.pdf (accessed on 29 April 2020).
9. Duarte, T.M.; Carinhas, N.; Barreiro, L.C.; Carrondo, M.J.; Alves, P.M.; Teixeira, A.P. Metabolic responses of CHO cells to limitation of key amino acids. *Biotechnol. Bioeng.* **2014**, *111*, 2095–2106. [CrossRef]
10. Crowell, C.K.; Grampp, G.E.; Rogers, G.N.; Miller, J.; Scheinman, R.I. Amino acid and manganese supplementation modulates the glycosylation state of erythropoietin in a CHO culture system. *Biotechnol. Bioeng.* **2007**, *96*, 538–549. [CrossRef]
11. Zalai, D.; Hevér, H.; Lovász, K.; Molnár, D.; Wechselberger, P.; Hofer, A.; Párta, L.; Putics, Á.; Herwig, C. A control strategy to investigate the relationship between specific productivity and high-mannose glycoforms in CHO cells. *Appl. Microbiol. Biotechnol.* **2016**, *100*, 7011–7024. [CrossRef]

12. Hofer, A.; Herwig, C. Quantitative determination of nine water-soluble vitamins in the complex matrix of corn steep liquor for raw material quality assessment. *J. Chem. Technol. Biotechnol.* **2017**, *92*, 2106–2113. [CrossRef]
13. Hofer, A.; Hauer, S.; Kroll, P.; Fricke, J.; Herwig, C. In-depth characterization of the raw material corn steep liquor and its bioavailability in bioprocesses of Penicillium chrysogenum. *Process Biochem.* **2018**, *70*, 20–28. [CrossRef]
14. Bhatia, H.; Mehdizadeh, H.; Drapeau, D.; Yoon, S. In-line monitoring of amino acids in mammalian cell cultures using raman spectroscopy and multivariate chemometrics models. *Eng. Life Sci.* **2018**, *18*, 55–61. [CrossRef]
15. Larson, T.M.; Gawlitzek, M.; Evans, H.; Albers, U.; Cacia, J. Chemometric evaluation of on-line high-pressure liquid chromatography in mammalian cell cultures: Analysis of amino acids and glucose. *Biotechnol. Bioeng.* **2002**, *77*, 553–563. [CrossRef]
16. Cimander, C.; Mandenius, C.-F. Online monitoring of a bioprocess based on a multi-analyser system and multivariate statistical process modelling. *J. Chem. Technol. Biotechnol.* **2002**, *77*, 1157–1168. [CrossRef]
17. Van de Merbel, N.C.; Lingeman, H.; Brinkman, U.A. Sampling and analytical strategies in on-line bioprocess monitoring and control. *J. Chromatogr. A* **1996**, *725*, 13–27. [CrossRef]
18. Esmonde-White, K.A.; Cuellar, M.; Uerpmann, C.; Lenain, B.; Lewis, I.R. Raman spectroscopy as a process analytical technology for pharmaceutical manufacturing and bioprocessing. *Anal. Bioanal. Chem.* **2017**, *409*, 637–649. [CrossRef]
19. Lee, H.L.T.; Boccazzi, P.; Gorret, N.; Ram, R.J.; Sinskey, A.J. In situ bioprocess monitoring of Escherichia coli bioreactions using Raman spectroscopy. *Vib. Spectrosc.* **2004**, *35*, 131–137. [CrossRef]
20. Müller, J.; Knop, K.; Wirges, M.; Kleinebudde, P. Validation of Raman spectroscopic procedures in agreement with ICH guideline Q2 with considering the transfer to real time monitoring of an active coating process. *J. Pharm. Biomed. Anal.* **2010**, *53*, 884–894. [CrossRef]
21. Borys, M.C.; Linzer, D.I.H.; Papoutsakis, E.T. Culture pH affects expression rates and glycosylation of recombinant mouse placental lactogen proteins by Chinese hamster ovary (CHO) cells. *Biotechnology* **1993**, *11*, 720–724. [CrossRef] [PubMed]
22. Kim, S.H.; Lee, G.M. Differences in optimal pH and temperature for cell growth and antibody production between two Chinese hamster ovary clones derived from the same parental clone. *J. Microbiol. Biotechnol.* **2007**, *17*, 712–720. [PubMed]
23. Yoon, S.K.; Choi, S.L.; Song, J.Y.; Lee, G.M. Effect of culture pH on erythropoietin production by Chinese hamster ovary cells grown in suspension at 32.5 and 37.0 °C. *Biotechnol. Bioeng.* **2005**, *89*, 345–356. [CrossRef] [PubMed]
24. Franco, R.; Daniela, G.; Fabrizio, M.; Ilaria, G.; Detlev, H. Influence of osmolarity and pH increase to achieve a reduction of monoclonal antibodies aggregates in a production process. *Cytotechnology* **1999**, *29*, 11–25. [CrossRef] [PubMed]
25. Birch, J.R.; Racher, A.J. Antibody production. *Adv. Drug. Deliv.* **2006**, *58*, 671–685. [CrossRef] [PubMed]
26. Kroll, P.; Stelzer, I.V.; Herwig, C. Soft sensor for monitoring biomass subpopulations in mammalian cell culture processes. *Biotechnol. Lett.* **2017**, *39*, 1667–1673. [CrossRef] [PubMed]

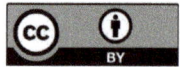

© 2020 by the authors. Licensee MDPI, Basel, Switzerland. This article is an open access article distributed under the terms and conditions of the Creative Commons Attribution (CC BY) license (http://creativecommons.org/licenses/by/4.0/).

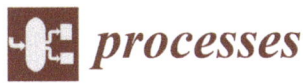

Article

High-Throughput Raman Spectroscopy Combined with Innovate Data Analysis Workflow to Enhance Biopharmaceutical Process Development

Stephen Goldrick [1,2,*,†], Alexandra Umprecht [3,*,†], Alison Tang [3], Roman Zakrzewski [1,2], Matthew Cheeks [2], Richard Turner [3], Aled Charles [3], Karolina Les [3], Martyn Hulley [3], Chris Spencer [2] and Suzanne S. Farid [1]

1. The Advanced Centre of Biochemical Engineering, Department of Biochemical Engineering, University College London, Gordon Street, London WC1E 6BT, UK; roman.zakrzewski@ucl.ac.uk (R.Z.); s.farid@ucl.ac.uk (S.S.F.)
2. Cell Culture & Fermentation Science, Biopharmaceuticals Development, R&D, AstraZeneca, Cambridge CB21 6GH, UK; matthew.cheeks@astrazeneca.com (M.C.); Spencerc@medimmune.com (C.S.)
3. Purification Process Sciences, Biopharmaceuticals Development, R&D, AstraZeneca, Cambridge CB21 6GH, UK; alison.tang@astrazeneca.com (A.T.); richard.turner@astrazeneca.com (R.T.); aled.charles@astrazeneca.com (A.C.); karolina.les@astrazeneca.com (K.L.); martyn.hulley@astrazeneca.com (M.H.)
* Correspondence: s.goldrick@ucl.ac.uk (S.G.); alexandra.umprecht@astrazeneca.com (A.U.); Tel.: +44-(0)-20-7679-0438 (S.G.)
† Both authors contributed equally to this work.

Received: 11 August 2020; Accepted: 10 September 2020; Published: 17 September 2020

Abstract: Raman spectroscopy has the potential to revolutionise many aspects of biopharmaceutical process development. The widespread adoption of this promising technology has been hindered by the high cost associated with individual probes and the challenge of measuring low sample volumes. To address these issues, this paper investigates the potential of an emerging new high-throughput (HT) Raman spectroscopy microscope combined with a novel data analysis workflow to replace off-line analytics for upstream and downstream operations. On the upstream front, the case study involved the at-line monitoring of an HT micro-bioreactor system cultivating two mammalian cell cultures expressing two different therapeutic proteins. The spectra generated were analysed using a partial least squares (PLS) model. This enabled the successful prediction of the glucose, lactate, antibody, and viable cell density concentrations directly from the Raman spectra without reliance on multiple off-line analytical devices and using only a single low-volume sample (50–300 µL). However, upon the subsequent investigation of these models, only the glucose and lactate models appeared to be robust based upon their model coefficients containing the expected Raman vibrational signatures. On the downstream front, the HT Raman device was incorporated into the development of a cation exchange chromatography step for an Fc-fusion protein to compare different elution conditions. PLS models were derived from the spectra and were found to predict accurately monomer purity and concentration. The low molecular weight (LMW) and high molecular weight (HMW) species concentrations were found to be too low to be predicted accurately by the Raman device. However, the method enabled the classification of samples based on protein concentration and monomer purity, allowing a prioritisation and reduction in samples analysed using A280 UV absorbance and high-performance liquid chromatography (HPLC). The flexibility and highly configurable nature of this HT Raman spectroscopy microscope makes it an ideal tool for bioprocess research and development, and is a cost-effective solution based on its ability to support a large range of unit operations in both upstream and downstream process operations.

Keywords: Raman spectroscopy; mammalian cell culture; process analytical technology; high-throughput; scale-down technologies; cation exchange chromatography; monitoring

1. Introduction

Process analytical technology (PAT) has been a major talking point within the biopharmaceutical sector since the release of the FDA's guidance for industry on PAT in 2004 [1]. The guidance encouraged a shift away from a fixed process that could result in product quality deviations towards an adaptive process ensuring a consistent product quality through sensors supporting advanced control strategies. Although there has been significant progress made towards achieving this goal, commercial manufacturing still heavily relies upon laborious off-line analytics and rudimentary control strategies. A major issue is the disconnect between early-stage research and development (R&D) activities and late-stage commercial manufacturing operations within the therapeutic drug lifecycle. These operations differ widely in terms of scale, where R&D operations utilise small volumes in the range of µL to L and commercial manufacturing processes operate with volumes in the range of 500 to 20,000 L. This large-scale difference can limit the universal application of a proposed PAT technology in the early stages of the drug development pipeline, therefore reducing the adoption of these core technologies within late-stage process development and commercialisation. To help bridge this gap, this paper focuses on the application of multivariate data analysis (MVDA) to better leverage at-line spectral measurements generated by a novel Raman spectroscopy microscope and utilise this information to support research and development (R&D) activities within the biopharmaceutical sector.

1.1. PAT for Upstream Processing

1.1.1. USP Monitoring and Analytics

Therapeutic proteins are highly complex and fragile molecules, and any upstream process deviations can lead to changes in the physiochemical, biological, and immunogenic properties of the molecule [2]. Therefore, controlling the bioreactor micro-environment is of paramount importance to ensure the product heterogeneity remains within a predefined specification defined by commercial good manufacturing practice (GMP) operations. To support this objective, the bioreactor is monitored and controlled through three classes of measurements, defined as on-line/in-line, at-line, or off-line [3]. The physical environment within the bioreactor, which includes the pH, temperature, and dissolved oxygen, utilises accurate and well-established on-line measurements with minimum time delays, enabling the real-time control of these variables. At-line and off-line monitoring involves removing a physical sample from the bioreactor for measurement in a separate analyser, enabling the monitoring of the chemical and biochemical environment. At-line measurements infer the close proximity of the analyser to the bioreactor, resulting in a shorter delay in the measurement availability, ranging from minutes to hours, whereas off-line measurements involve longer delay times of up to a day or even a week, depending on the analyser and delay before processing the sample. The traditional monitoring of upstream processing (USP) activities requires three different analysers: The first is an at-line biochemical analyser that measures the daily metabolite concentrations, including glucose and lactate, and typically takes between 5 and 10 min per sample. The second is an at-line cell counter that measures the cell densities and viabilities every 1 or 2 days with an analysis time of 5–10 min per sample. The third analyser is an off-line protein A HPLC column that measures the protein concentration and product quality; this is the slowest analytical device, as the sample needs to be purified before loading onto the column, and these measurements are typically only available after the experiment is complete. The manual sampling procedure and slow response time of these analysers limit the ability of these measurements to be used for control strategies. The additional drawback of these traditional methods is that they are destructive and therefore require separate samples for each analyser.

A recent report targeting the biopharmaceutical industry has identified and prioritised the top bioreactor variables requiring investment in at-line/in-line monitoring technologies to facilitate effective in-process control strategies [4]. This priority list includes the cell viability, viable cell density (VCD), glucose concentration, amino acids, and product concentration, defined as the bioreactor's critical process parameters (CPPs), in addition to the glycosylation profile and charge profile, defined as the critical quality attributes (CQAs). These variables are all currently measured by slow and laborious off-line analytical analysers. PAT aims to change the reliance of biopharmaceutical companies on these slow off-line analytical measurements.

1.1.2. PAT within USP Mammalian Cell Cultures

PAT ultimately aims to integrate aspects of chemical, physical, microbiological, mathematical, and risk analyses to ensure robust biopharmaceutical operation [5]. There are various on-line and in-line PAT technologies suitable for USP mammalian cell culture monitoring. Capacitance sensors have gained popularity recently and provide robust measurements of viable cell density. These probes measure the radio frequency impedance in the cell broth and can distinguish between live and dead cells based on the assumption of living cells having intact spherical cell walls. Konakovsky et al. demonstrated the ability of capacitance probes to accurately predict VCD for mammalian cell cultures using a robust partial least squares (PLS) model that could be transferred between clones and across scales [6]. The majority of other PATs are spectroscopic, and are advantageous due to their ability to measure multiple components within the bioreactor. Examples include infrared spectroscopy, which measures reflectance, transflectance, and transmission events during near-infrared (NIR) or mid-infrared (MIR) irradiation. NIR was demonstrated by Hakemeyer et al. to predict numerous mammalian cell culture variables, including the cell viability, product concentration, glucose, and lactate, with the predictions validated across multiple scales, ranging from 2.5 to 1000 L [7]. Additionally, Sandor et al. compared the ability of NIR and MIR for mammalian cell monitoring and concluded that MIR has a higher accuracy for individual analyte concentrations, such as glucose and lactate, but recommended NIR as a better tool for the on-line monitoring of mammalian cell systems based on its ability to measure cell densities through light scattering effects, which is not possible with MIR excitation [8]. Ultraviolet and visible spectroscopy is another tool and one of the oldest forms of spectroscopy based upon the Beer–Lambert law. However, this technology has limited demonstrations within USP which have primarily focused on predicting the total cell density, as shown by Ude et al. [9]. Fluorescence spectroscopy is another valuable tool that takes advantage of the fluorescence nature of many biological components excited by visible or UV light. Typically, within mammalian cell cultures, 2D fluorescence spectroscopy is employed. Ohadi et al. demonstrated the ability of this technique to predict numerous variables, including the product concentration and glucose, and also to distinguish between living and dead cells, therefore making it an attractive tool for the in situ monitoring of mammalian cell cultures [10]. Another major advantage of this technology is the ability to exploit the auto-fluorescence nature of various variables, such as amino acids, vitamins, and proteins, including selected molecules or targets tagged using fluorescence markers. Calvet et al. used a type of fluorescence spectroscopy called Excitation Emission Matrix spectroscopy to generate a three-dimensional contour plot of the excitation wavelength vs. emission wavelength vs. fluorescence. The method generates accurate fingerprints for multicomponent systems and was demonstrated by Calvet et al. to identify the composition changes of tryptophan and tyrosine in a complex media applicable to industrial mammalian cell cultures [11]. The primary benefit of these spectroscopic tools is that they are non-destructive, non-invasive, and highly informative, making them highly suitable for mammalian cell culture monitoring.

1.1.3. Applications of Raman Spectroscopy in USP

In comparison to other spectroscopic methods, Raman spectroscopy has gained attention in recent years due to its suitability for the analysis of aqueous samples due to its low water interference and high specificity. Raman spectroscopy excites the sample using a monochromatic light source, causing small vibrational frequency shifts in the sample. The inelastic scattering of this light source generates Raman spectra containing quantitative and qualitative information, including the composition, chemical environment, and structural information related to the sample. The major challenge with Raman spectroscopy is the low signal to noise ratio due to the weak Raman scattering signals compared to the incident wavelength. These weak signals can be corrupted by strong fluorescence signals associated with the analysis of biological samples [12]. Alternative methods such as Surface Enhanced Raman Spectroscopy (SERS) have been developed to overcome these issues. Different types of Raman Spectroscopy, including Resonance Raman Spectroscopy, Raman Optical Activity, and surface-enhanced Raman spectroscopy (SERS), as well as their applications, are extensively described in a review by Buckley and Ryder [13].

Within USP, the biopharmaceutical industry has focused on Raman spectroscopy as one of the leading PAT technologies to monitor fermentation systems cultivating different expression systems, such as bacterial [14], fungal [12], and mammalian cell culture systems, including NS0 and HEK293 cell lines [15,16]. However, the majority of Raman spectroscopy monitoring operations focus on Chinese hamster ovary (CHO) mammalian cell lines, and have demonstrated the ability of this technology to predict the previously prioritised CPPs of glucose, lactate, VCD, and product concentration [15,17,18]. The proven ability to monitor these variables has led to the development of adaptive control strategies, as demonstrated by Craven et al., who applied a nonlinear model predictive controller to maintain the glucose concentration of a mammalian cell culture at a fixed set-point [19]. Additional control demonstrations include the application of a closed-loop control strategy using in-line Raman spectroscopy to minimise lactate accumulation through glucose feed rate additions, which resulted in the additional benefit of increasing the product concentration by approximately 85% [15]. More recently, Raman spectroscopy has shown promise as a replacement tool for the pH control of mammalian cell cultures [20]. However, the feasibility of this is questionable, given the relatively long acquisition time of each Raman spectra, which was between 16 and 20 min, in comparison to traditional pH probes with a response time of seconds. Raman spectroscopy has also been used to monitor the glycosylation patterns of a monoclonal antibody, which, as previously discussed, is a high-priority CQA. Li at al. utilised Raman spectroscopy for the real-time monitoring of a monoclonal antibody, and were able to distinguish between glycosylated and non-glycosylated molecules [21]. The ability to monitor product quality in real-time opens up significant opportunities for USP optimisation and advanced feedback control solutions.

1.2. PAT for Downstream Processing (DSP)

1.2.1. DSP Monitoring and Analytics of Mammalian Therapeutic Products

Typical PAT for downstream processing predominantly includes various sensors for the single-variable monitoring of CPPs. These include pH and conductivity probes, pressure and flow rate sensors, and UV spectroscopic measurements and other sensors, which are analysed through means of univariate analysis and/or operator knowledge. Additional information, especially regarding the CQAs of the product, is obtained through off-line analysis, which allows the determination of process and product-related quality attributes. Whereas univariate monitoring is suitable for the monitoring of process variables, it rarely carries enough information to be able to measure CQAs such as product multimers; product charge variants; host cell-related impurities, such as host cell proteins (HCPs), DNA, and lipids, in addition to impurities such as resin leachables. CQAs are monitored using univariate off-line/at-line analytical techniques, with efforts being made to enable online implementation.

Multiple-antibody CQAs, such as the high molecular weight (HMW) and low molecular weight (LMW) species content, charge, and glycosylation variants, are most commonly performed utilising at-line/off-line HPLC utilising various column chemistries, including size-exclusion (SE-HPLC) and ion-exchange (IEX-HPLC) liquid chromatography. In SE-HPLC, different-sized product species are separated based on their differential retention time, and content percentages are calculated as the area under curve (AUC) for peaks corresponding to the UV absorption signal of the elution product [22]. As standard SE-HPLC has long run times (commonly 20 min per sample), efforts have been made to increase the speed of analysis and implement SE-HPLC-based methods on-line [23]. Decreasing the time needed for sample analysis to less than 5 min was made possible by utilising ultra-high-performance liquid chromatography (UHPLC) with sub-2μm particles [24,25], and these approaches were further developed by coupling to mass spectroscopy [26]. Alternative approaches to UHPLC were also described, such as membrane chromatography, with an analysis time as low as 1.5 min [27]. The real-time analysis of aggregates and charge variants during cation exchange (CEX) chromatography using HPLC has been described by Tiwari et al. [28]. Patel et al. describes the use of on-line UHPLC for the detection of charge variants in continuous processes, which can be adapted for aggregate analysis [29]. Although the feasibility of these approaches has been demonstrated, on-line HPLC/UHPLC has not yet been widely adopted.

Another important set of antibody product CQAs are host-related impurities, such as host cell proteins (HCPs), DNA, and lipids; and process-related impurities, such as free protein A ligands. HCPs and protein A ligands are typically detected through various immunological assays, including traditional ELISA and high-throughput microfluidic assays. The processing time can be decreased by moving from a traditional ELISA to an automated ELISA using liquid-handling systems and automated microfluidic systems [30]; these still do not allow real-time analysis, as the time needed to run these assays is in the order of hours. Efforts have been made to develop immunological methods capable of on-line measurements utilising a flow cell, although the analysis time of above 30 min per sample would not suit the current downstream requirements [31]. As the system described in Kumar et al. was developed for upstream applications with lower requirements for time of analysis, additional changes to the systems, such as parallel flow cells, could potentially be made to enable Downstream Processing (DSP) application.

Although there has been progress in adapting traditional at-line methods to allow real-time control, most methods still suffer from long run times. In order to expand process control and enable the real-time monitoring of CQAs, multivariate approaches and PAT are necessary.

1.2.2. Applications of PAT in DSP

Various spectroscopic methods, including infra-red (IR), mid-IR (MIR), Raman, Fourier-transform IR, fluorescence, and UV spectroscopy, have been applied to downstream processing. As described extensively in a review by Rudt. et al. [32], and more recently in Rolinger et al. [33], each of these spectroscopic techniques has its own set of advantages and applications.

Examples of spectroscopic methods applied to DSP monitoring include the use of UV-spectroscopy with PLS modelling to automatically control the loading phase of protein A chromatography by monitoring the concentration of the monoclonal antibody (mAb) product in the load [34]. UV spectroscopy has been also shown to monitor mAb aggregate and monomer concentrations [35], although during the investigated runs the monomer and aggregate peaks showed a good separation, which might not always be the case and could decrease the otherwise high sensitivity of predictions. These studies benefited from the utilisation of variable pathlength spectroscopym enabling accurate in-line measurements even at high concentrations. The same device was recently applied to the on-line monitoring of ultrafiltration/diafiltration (UF/DF) as part of a multi-sensor PAT capable of monitoring concentration in addition to the apparent molecular weight using dynamic light scattering (DLS) to monitor changes in aggregation during the process [36].

Other spectroscopic methods have been described in relation to DSP, such as mid (MIR) and near (NIR) infrared spectroscopy. NIR was used to determine mAb concentration in real-time, enabling the dynamic loading of protein A chromatography [37]. Capito et al. used MIR to monitor product concentration, aggregate, and HCP content, although this was developed as an at-line method, as the samples were processed (dried) prior to measurements [38], limiting the use of the tool for on-line monitoring. Additionally, there have been attempts to overcome the limitations of individual spectral techniques by integrating multiple different inputs. In a study by Walch et al., standard detectors

(UV, pH, conductivity) were implemented alongside additional techniques including fluorescence spectroscopy, MIR, light scattering, and refractive index measurement to monitor the protein A chromatography. These inputs were then analysed through PLS regression, producing predictive models for mAb concentration, monomer purity, aggregate content, and host related impurities (HCPs, DNA). This has resulted in accurate predictions for titre and monomer purity, but less so for HCPs, DNA, and % aggregate, especially when the sample matrix was changed [39].

1.2.3. Applications of Raman Spectroscopy in DSP

The applications of Raman spectroscopy in DSP include the measurement of product concentration, product aggregation, glycosylation, and membrane fouling. Predicting the product concentration of mAb was first shown by Andre et al. using an immersion probe [40], and further expanded by Feidl et al. through the development of a Raman flow cell [41,42]. Determining the titre is especially relevant for continuous perfusion processes, as it allows the dynamic loading of subsequent capture steps, as demonstrated in [43]. However, the titre determination from harvest can arguably be achieved by the use of delta UV spectroscopy comparing the A280 absorbance of the feed and eluate [44], which might be easier to implement as it does not require MVDA modelling. Therefore, if Raman spectroscopy is to be widely adopted in DSP, it must provide additional information.

There are studies demonstrating the ability of Raman spectroscopy to distinguish between samples with a high content of aggregate mAb species. Typically, these studies are performed at high mAb concentrations and/or high aggregate contents for the purpose of proof-of-concept studies, in addition to studies of aggregation in the formulated drug products. Zhou et al. monitored the thermally induced aggregation of intravenous IgG (IVIG) at high concentrations (51 mg/mL), describing the various spectral features present upon aggregation, in particular shift in the tyrosine peak at 830 and 850 cm^{-1} and the tryptophan peak at 1550 cm^{-1} for the IVIG, using Raman spectroscopy coupled with DLS [45]. Thermally induced aggregation was described in another study, where five antibodies with various propensities to aggregate were analysed using the perturbation-correlation moving windows method, visualising changes in the spectra during heating. By studying multiple different mAbs, differences were observed in the aggregation mechanism and associated spectral features [46], which might potentially make it difficult to develop models that could be utilised across multiple antibody formats. The presence of subtle differences in the sequence and structure of mAbs resulting in significantly different spectra is further supported by a study using SERS for the label-free identification of different antibody products by PLS-DA [47]. Although not explicitly described in the study, the described spectral differences might not only stem from the varying structural features, but also from the composition of the formulation buffer, product concentration, etc., for which the study did not adjust. In order to utilise Raman spectroscopy for aggregate analysis, quantitative predictive models are needed. Initial steps towards such models are described by Zhan et al., where mixtures of HMW and monomer were used to generate a model, which was then validated with independent samples generated through incubation at 40 °C. The model was able to predict the validation samples with a root mean square error of prediction (RMSEP) of 1.8% [48]. To monitor HMW and LMW species during chromatography runs, the methods need to be sensitive enough to allow detection at relevant concentrations (<10 mg/mL) and low aggregate contents (<10%). In all the above-mentioned studies, the samples typically had either high concentrations and/or high aggregate contents, which might not make these models suitable for the monitoring of standard preparative chromatography. Furthermore, the models need to be robust enough to deal with the changing background of co-eluting impurities and changes in buffer composition, which is common in gradient elution and is yet to be described.

Other CQAs might also have a potential to be monitored by Raman spectroscopy. Spectral differences in antibody glycosylation have been described in simple systems (glycosylated vs. non glycosylated proteins) [49–51], suggesting potential for elucidating more subtle differences in glycosylation that are relevant to bioprocessing. Another interesting area that could be investigated using Raman spectroscopy is the detection of HCPs, for which there are currently no published studies.

Early efforts have been made using FT-IR by Capito et al. with limited sensitivity [52], which does not allow for widespread use. Overall, detecting HCPs might require more complex approaches, such as Raman labels, since HCPs are a structurally diverse group of proteins and therefore lack a distinct Raman signature.

Raman spectroscopy can also be utilised in process monitoring. Virtanen et al. describes using Raman spectroscopy in membrane fouling monitoring, where an immersion probe was placed into a cross-flow filtration unit, and fouling over time by vanillin, a model organic foulant, was monitored using PCA [53]. The applicability of this approach to DSP needs to be evaluated separately using relevant molecules, as potential issues might include the weaker signal of proteins compared to small organic molecules, as well as the more complex background matrix.

Overall, the application of Raman spectroscopy to DSP is a relatively young field and is expected to be further advanced in the future, as innovations in instrumentation as well as advanced techniques such as SERS become available and widely implemented.

1.3. High-Throughput Raman Spectroscopy and Its Advantages for Bioprocess Development

The acquisition set-up and type of system utilised in Raman spectroscopy typically depends on the application and on whether it requires at-line or in-line/on-line measurement. Common set-ups include immersion probes, flow cells, single cuvette systems, microscope slides, and high-throughput systems. Here, we present a high-throughput Raman spectroscopy microscope based on standard 96-well plates, which allows combined use for both upstream and downstream development.

Raman spectroscopy in USP is commonly based on an optic fibre immersion probe for each bioreactor, although multiple probes can be connected to a single Raman spectrometer. Alternatively, HT scale-down models such as ambr^{TM} 15 (Sartorius Stedim, Göttingen, Germany) with at-line (Rowland-Jones and Jaques 2019) or integrated Raman measurement can be utilised for model building, although the latter has only been introduced recently. These systems work well for upstream applications, but might lack versatility to allow their use in other areas of bioprocess development.

An alternative approach is the use of a high-throughput Raman device which is suitable for model generation for both upstream and downstream applications. The HT Raman devices described in the literature include commercial devices such as the RamanRxn1™ High Throughput Screener (HTS) (Kaiser Optical Systems, Ann Arbor, MI, USA) [54], the InVia confocal microscope (Renishaw, Wotton-under-Edge, UK) presented in this work, the Lab Ram HR Evolution confocal microscope (Horiba Jobin Yvon, Kyoto, Japan) [55], and custom-built devices assembled using parts from various manufacturers [56,57]. Data acquisition is performed using well plates, typically 96-well plates, however settings can be adjusted to allow acquisition for other high-throughput labware or bespoke applications. Automatic plate mapping allows autonomous operation, allowing the screening of a large number of samples.

Whereas using HT Raman is more laborious when coupled with standard bioreactors requiring manual sampling, it is highly suitable for experiments using scale-down micro-bioreactors, where sampling is typically automated. A major advantage of these systems is the small sample requirement equal to 50–100 µL that is necessary for a measurement enabling the primary CPPs and CQAs to be predicted. This reduces the reliance on multiple analysers, thus reducing the capital and operational costs while providing near real-time information on difficult-to-monitor variables such as product concentration. Similarly, HT Raman is also suitable for model building in DSP. Samples can be generated through elution fractionation during preparative chromatography, where fractionating into a standardised labware minimises the number of manual steps.

The research outlined in this paper investigates the predictive capabilities of an HT Raman microscope combined with advanced data analytics to support both USP and DSP research and development operations. The paper demonstrates the ability of this technology to monitor the CPPs within an HT microbioreactor system in addition to monitoring monomer and product concentration within the development of a CEX chromatography step. At the core of these activities is the application of MVDA models to convert these multiple-dimensional spectral data sets into quantitative information necessary for monitoring. This involved negating the influence of corrupting fluorescence through baseline and scattering correction algorithms, in addition to the evaluation of the models' coefficients, enabling more robustness in predictive models. In summary, this technology was found to be highly versatile and applicable across a wide range of unit operations in bioprocess development, provided the correct MVDA models are implemented.

2. Materials and Methods

2.1. Product Materials

Three different molecules were used in this study; in the USP experiments, cell line A produced an antibody-peptide fusion protein, and cell line B produced a modified IgG1 molecule. In the DSP study, an Fc-fusion protein was investigated. All the molecules utilised in this work were developed internally and provided by AstraZeneca, Cambridge, UK.

2.2. Cell Line and Cell Culture Propagation

Cell line A and cell line B in the USP work, and the cell line utilised in the DSP work, used a Chinese hamster ovary (CHO) host expressing high levels of therapeutic protein. These cell lines were provided by AstraZeneca and are proprietary and commercial products. No human cells were involved in this work. The cell lines were cultivated in chemically defined CHO media, maintained at 37 °C under 5% carbon dioxide, shaken at a constant rpm, and passaged 2–3 times per week for propagation and scale-up for inoculation.

2.3. Bioreactor Systems and Cell Culture Process

Two cell lines were cultivated in an advanced micro-bioreactor (ambr^{TM} 15) system (Sartorius Stedim) with 24 single vessels split into two separate culture stations, where each vessel was operated with a 11–15 mL working volume. Cell line A was cultivated in vessels 1–12, and cell line B was cultivated in vessels 13–24. The experimental set-up investigated the impact of both different dissolved oxygen (DO_2) set-points in addition to DO_2 fluctuations on both cellular growth and protein production. The DO_2 set-point was controlled to 40% and was fluctuated every 15 min to either 10% or 20% by purging with nitrogen. For cell line A, vessels 1 and 2 were maintained at a DO_2 set-point of 40%, vessels 3 and 9 were controlled to 10%, and vessels 3 and 10 were controlled to 20%. Vessels 5 and 11 were fluctuated between 40–10%, and vessels 6, 7, 11, and 12 were fluctuated between 40% and 20%. Cell line B followed the same experimental set-up as cell line A for vessels 13–24. The temperature and pH of all the vessels was controlled to 35.5 °C and 7, respectively, and the agitation rate was adjusted to ensure that the DO_2 concentration set-points were maintained. The feeding strategy involved five equally spaced additions of the feed after the initial feed day indicated. The initial seeding density was <10 × 10^5 cells mL^{-1}. The culture pH was controlled to 7 through the addition of sodium carbonate and sparging with CO_2 gas, with its control strategy implementing a pH dead-band equal to 0.1. Antifoam volumes of 20 µL were added as required. Daily at-line samples were analysed for the glucose and lactate concentrations using the 2950D Biochemistry Analyser (YSI, Yellow Springs, OH, USA) and every second day for the viable cell density (VCD) and viability using the Vi-Cell Automated cell viability analyser (Beckman Coulter, Brea, CA, USA).

2.4. Titre Analysis

Volumetric antibody-peptide fusion titres in cell culture supernatants were quantified by protein A affinity chromatography using a protein A ImmunoDetection sensor cartridge (Applied Biosystems, Warrington, UK) coupled with an Agilent 1200 series HPLC (Agilent, Berkshire, UK). Peak areas relative to a reference standard calibration curve were used to calculate the titres. These samples were measured on days 2, 4, 6, 8, and 10 for the ambrTM 15 system.

2.5. CEX Sample Generation

The Fc-fusion protein used in the DSP part of this study was generated using a CHO host provided by AstraZeneca, UK, Cambridge. Chromatographic experiments were carried out using an ÄKTA Avant controlled with Unicorn Software version 7.1 (Cytiva, Marlborough, MA, USA). The protein feed was purified using MabSelect Sure Protein A chromatography resin (Cytiva, Marlborough, MA, USA), subjected to a low-pH treatment, and purified further using CaptoAdhere resins (Cytiva, Marlborough, MA, USA) in flow-through mode. Screening experiments were conducted to determine the optimal conditions to purify fusion proteins on Poros 50 HS resin (Thermo Fisher Scientific, Bedford, MA) using varying conditions of the elution buffer. The elution was performed either in gradient mode from 0–0.5 M of NaCl in 20 mM of sodium citrate or step mode using 20 mM of sodium citrate (for calibration set (T1) and validation set 1 (P1)) and 50 mM of sodium citrate (for validation set 2 (P2)) with NaCl in the range 133–210 mM, at a pH range of 5.8–6.2 and a loading concentration of 10–20 g/L. The elution was fractionated into 1 mL fractions, where each fraction constituted a separate sample for spectral measurements.

2.6. Protein Concentration and Analytical Size Exclusion Chromatography

Sample concentration was determined off-line by A280 UV spectrometry using Trinean (Unchained Labs, Pleasanton, CA, USA) with the corresponding extinction coefficient. Only samples with a product concentration above 0.5 mg/mL were used for the Raman measurements. The monomer purity was monitored with high-performance size exclusion chromatography (HP-SEC) using a TSK-GEL G3000SWXL column (7.8 mm × 30 cm) from Tosoh Bioscience (King of Prussia, PA, USA) with an Agilent 1200 HPLC system (Agilent Technologies, Santa Clara, CA, USA). The column was operated at a flow rate of 1 mL/min with a mobile phase consisting of 0.1 M of sodium phosphate and 0.1 M of sodium sulphate, pH 6.8. Protein was monitored by the absorbance at 280 nm, and the sample purity was estimated by integrating the chromatograms.

2.7. Spectral Data Acquisition

All the spectral measurements were performed using the InVia confocal Raman microscope (Renishaw, Wotton-under-Edge, UK) equipped with a 785 nm laser. Prior to spectral measurements, the acquisition settings were optimised in respect to the focal point, sample volume, laser output, and duration of measurements. Measurements of the cell culture were performed in the range of 381 to 1534 cm^{-1} using a 10% laser power (30 mW), 30 s acquisition time, 5 accumulations, and line-focus using a 5X objective (Leica Microsystems, Wetzlar, Germany). For each sample, 350 µL of culture was spun down to remove cells, and 300 µL of supernatant was used for the acquisition. The data acquisition was performed using polypropylene (PP) 96-well plates (Greiner Bio-one, Stonehouse, UK) using the Microplate mapping option of the WiRe 5.2 software (Renishaw, Wotton-under-Edge, UK). Data acquisition for the CEX samples was performed similarly to the cell culture samples, with a difference in acquisition range (605–1741 cm^{-1}). Additional experiments were performed comparing the signal from the PP 96-well plates with the signal from stainless steel plates, which were custom-made. The acquisition was further optimised using a long-distance 50X objective (Leica Microsystems, Wetzlar, Germany), increasing the laser power to 100%, and decreasing the acquisition time to 10 s and 3 accumulations.

2.8. Spectral Data Pre-Processing and Model Set-Up

The Raman data recorded by the HT InVia Raman microscope for both the USP and DSP applications were pre-processed and modelled in Python 3.7.1. PLS was used to develop the predictions of the variables in both the USP and DSP case studies. In the analysis of the USP variables and the product concentration in the DSP case study, the background fluorescence was removed by fitting and subtracting a 1st order polynomial to each individual spectrum using the open-source

Rampy library [58] (Le Losq 2018). The baseline corrected spectra were subsequently normalised by applying a standard normal variate (SNV) algorithm, which corrects for scattering effects due to slight changes in the path length of the Raman device in addition to correcting for changes in the cell culture composite such as viscosity. Prior to the SNV, the data were smoothed using a Savitzky–Golay smoothing filter. For the monomer concentration in the DSP case study, the PLS model was developed using the raw spectra. In the USP application, the calibration data set consisted of cell cultures: 1–5 and 7–11 (cell line A), 13–17 and 19–23 (cell line B), and the validation runs equal to cell cultures 6 and 12 (cell line A) and 8 and 24 (cell line B). In the DSP application, the individual CEX runs differed in the elution buffer conditions, where the calibration set consisted of elution fractions from runs using 20 mM of sodium citrate, with varying levels of sodium chloride (0–0.5 M). There were two district validation sets—the first (P1) was in an identical buffer range to that of the calibration set and consisted of 40 samples, whereas the second (P2) consisted of elution fractions using elution buffer containing 50 mM of sodium citrate as well as a wider salt range (133–210 mM), and consisted of 22 samples. The optimum number of latent variables for each of the PLS models was identified by minimising both the root mean square error (RMSE) based on the calibration data set and the root mean square error of prediction (RMSEP) based on the validation data set.

2.9. Partial Least Squares Model Generation

The PLS model implemented the nonlinear iterative partial least squares (NIPALS) algorithm, as outlined in detail by Wold et al. [59]. The preprocessed spectral data ($X_{Spectra}$) were first decomposed into N latent variables, generating a matrix of scores, T, and loadings, P, with E as the residuals. The off-line concentration of the glucose concentration ($Y_{Variable}$) was decomposed in a similar fashion, generating a matrix of scores, U, and loadings, Q, with F as the residuals:

$$X_{Spectra} = TP^T + E, \tag{1}$$

$$Y_{Variable} = UQ^T + F. \tag{2}$$

The inner-relationship B vector is generated by relating the scores of the $X_{Spectra}$ to the scores of the $Y_{Variable}$, calculated as:

$$B = X_{Spectra}^T(T)\left(X_{Spectra}^T X_{Spectra}\right)^{-1}. \tag{3}$$

The PLS model works iteratively through each latent variable and, upon convergence, generates a matrix of regression coefficients β equal to:

$$\beta = W\left(P^T W\right)^{-1} diag(B). \tag{4}$$

The predicted Y variable ($\dot{Y}_{Variable}$) is calculated with the cumulative sum of the regression coefficients, taking N latent variables, defined by Goldrick et al. 2018 as [12]:

$$\dot{Y}_{Variable} = X_{Spectra} \sum_{n=1}^{N} \beta. \tag{5}$$

3. Results and Discussion

This paper evaluates the performance of a novel HT-Raman spectroscopy device applied to two critical USP and DSP operations within biopharmaceutical manufacturing. This evaluation includes the development of a Raman spectroscopy model generation workflow shown in Figure 1, outlining the necessary steps to ensure that a robust MVDA model is generated. The novelty of the presented workflow is that, in addition to quantifying the performance of the MVDA model using traditional RMSE and RMSEP metrics, it suggests interpreting the model's coefficients and comparing them to the expected Raman vibrational signatures of the variable investigated to ensure that the accuracy of the predictions are independent of the metabolism-induced concentration correlations. This novel Raman spectroscopy model generation workflow is demonstrated on two case studies, the first involves the at-line monitoring of an HT micro-bioreactor system cultivating two mammalian cells expressing two different therapeutic proteins. The second application of this device involves the development of a cation exchange chromatography step for an Fc-fusion protein to compare different elution conditions.

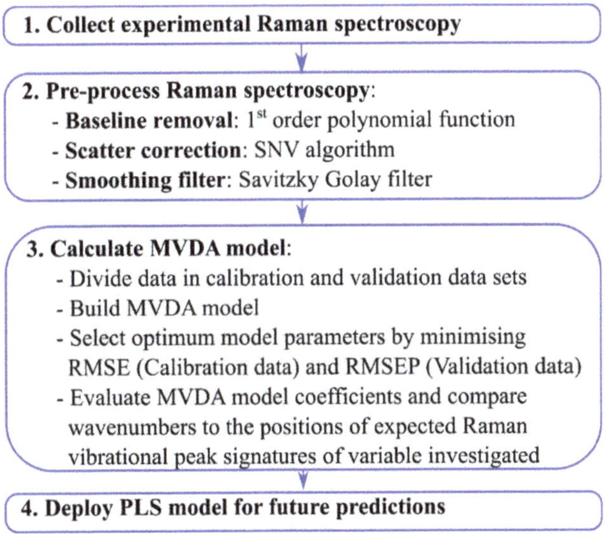

1. Collect experimental Raman spectroscopy

2. Pre-process Raman spectroscopy:
   - **Baseline removal**: 1st order polynomial function
   - **Scatter correction**: SNV algorithm
   - **Smoothing filter**: Savitzky Golay filter

3. Calculate MVDA model:
   - Divide data in calibration and validation data sets
   - Build MVDA model
   - Select optimum model parameters by minimising RMSE (Calibration data) and RMSEP (Validation data)
   - Evaluate MVDA model coefficients and compare wavenumbers to the positions of expected Raman vibrational peak signatures of variable investigated

4. Deploy PLS model for future predictions

Figure 1. Raman spectroscopy model generation workflow defining the primary steps to ensure that a robust MVDA model is generated. SNV = standard normal variate, RMSE = root mean square, and RMSEP = root mean square error of prediction, MVDA = multivariate data analysis.

3.1. Demonstration of HT Raman Spectroscopy Microscope to USP

In this work, the HT InVia Raman microscope was applied to two essential R&D unit operations within biopharmaceutical manufacturing. The first investigated the application of MVDA to transform the Raman spectra from a USP operation to predict the primary metabolite concentrations, cellular growth characteristics, and therapeutic protein concentrations of a mammalian cell culture performed on a micro-bioreactor system. The off-line variables investigated in this work were recorded every 48 h and are shown in Figure 2. In total, there were 12 cell culture runs from cell line A and 12 cell culture runs from cell line B, with the majority of these harvested early on day 10 due to the high accumulation of lactate, as shown in Figure 2C. The high lactate production was due to controlled fluctuations in the DO_2 set-point that involved manipulating the DO_2 to between 10–40% and studying the influence of these fluctuations on the growth and productivity. The adjustments to the DO_2 set-points resulted in the majority of the cells maintaining their lactate production state from day 4 to 10. The influence of these DO_2 concentration fluctuations on lactate production is outside the scope of this paper. Apart from the lactate concentration, the glucose, VCD, and antibody concentrations shown in Figure 2 represent the typical ranges expected for mammalian cell cultures, providing an ideal data set to investigate the performance of this HT-Raman spectroscopy device. The analysis of the experimental Raman spectra followed the workflow shown in Figure 1, and the MVDA model chosen was a PLS model defined by Section 2.9. The data split used to build this PLS model is shown in Figure 2, with runs 1–5 and 7–11 (cell line A) and 13–17 and 19–23 (cell line B) used for calibration, and runs 6 and 12 (cell line A) and 18 and 24 (cell line B) used for validation.

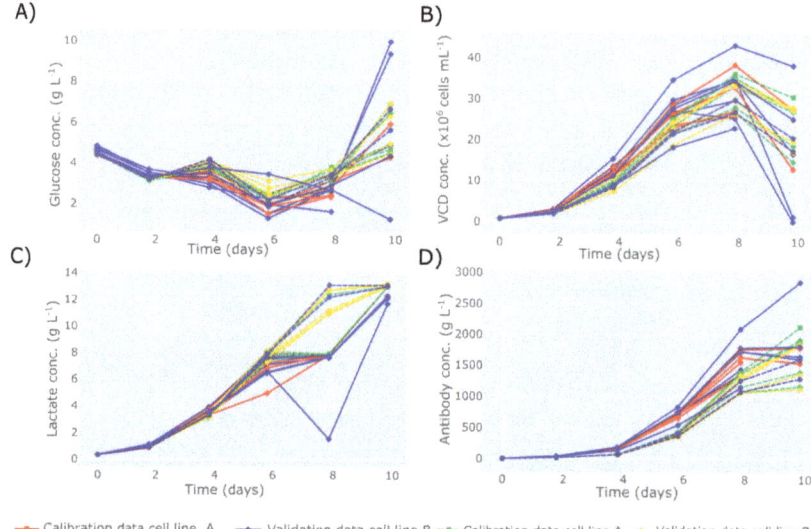

Figure 2. Time series plots of off-line analytics recorded on a micro-bioreactor system for (**A**) glucose concentration, (**B**) viable cell density (VCD) concentration, (**C**) lactate concentration, and (**D**) antibody concentration. Cell line A is indicated by the solid lines with the red lines and squares representing the calibration cell cultures: 1–5 and 7–11. The validation runs are indicated by the blue lines with diamonds, and represent cell cultures 6 and 12. Cell line B is indicated by the dashed lines with the green lines and squares representing the calibration cell cultures: 13–17 and 19–23. The validation runs are indicated by the yellow lines with diamonds and represent cell cultures 18 and 24. The micro-bioreactor system had 24 parallel bioreactors with an initial working volume of 13.5 mL, operated using a pH set-point of 7, DO_2 concentrations of between 10–40%, and a temperature maintained at 35.5 °C.

The spectral analysis was carried out using the remaining off-line analytic sample, equivalent to 300 µL. This material was split up into three separate wells on a 96-well plate, providing triplicate 100 µL samples for the HT InVia Raman microscope device. The selected sample volume of 100 µL was found to produce the most consistent spectra, although smaller volumes can be accommodated. The raw spectral data is shown in Figure 3A and highlights the significant baseline increase as the culture progresses from day 0 (inoculation) to day 10. An approximate 15-fold increase is observed in the average baseline of the Raman spectra recorded on day 0 compared to day 10. Corrupting fluorescence still remains a major problem for Raman spectroscopy, particularly during upstream processing operations, where broad fluorescence background signals have been shown to mask out important Raman peaks and thus prevent the extraction of useful correlations [12]. To minimise the influence of fluorescence in this work, a baseline removal algorithm was implemented, followed by the application of a scattering correction algorithm referred to as standard normal variate (SNV). The application of SNV is highly recommended when using a HT Raman spectroscopy microscope, as it corrects for minor path length differences between the laser source and the sample due to small volume changes, resulting in the baseline displacement of the spectrum along the vertical axis. These pre-processed spectral data are shown in Figure 3B and were used to develop the PLS models of glucose, VCD, lactate, and antibody concentrations. Alternative methods to remove strong fluorescence signals include taking the 1st derivate of the spectra, followed by SNV. This was demonstrated by Berry et al., who observed a significant baseline shift during the on-line monitoring of a CHO cell culture system and generated highly accurate models of multiple process parameters including glucose, lactate, and VCD (Berry et al. 2015).

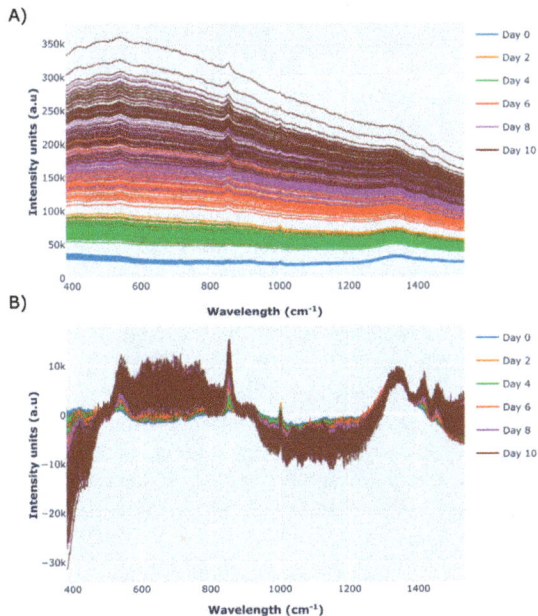

Figure 3. Raman spectra recorded by the high-throughput Raman spectroscopy microscope for each of the 24 micro-bioreactor cell culture runs on day 0–10 shown in the form of (**A**) the raw spectral data and (**B**) the baseline-corrected spectra, using a 1st order polynomial function followed by the application of a standard normal variate (SNV) scattering scatter algorithm and a Savitzky–Golay smoothing filter. Each spectrum was generated using 5 accumulations each with a 30 s acquisition time, recorded using 10% laser power (30 mW).

Four separate PLS models were developed to correlate the pre-processed spectra shown in Figure 3B to the concentrations of glucose and lactate, VCD, and the antibody concentration. The model was calibrated using cell culture runs 1–5 and 7–11 (cell line A) and 13–17 and 19–23 (cell line B), and validated with runs 6 and 12 (cell line A) and 18 and 24 (cell line B). The prediction performances of the optimum PLS models for each variable are summarised in Table 1. The choice of latent variables was based on minimising the root mean square error (RMSE) for the calibration data sets and the root mean square error of the prediction (RMSEP) values for the validation data sets, which ensured an accurate model with a good prediction performance. However, a low RMSE and RMSEP does not always equate to a robust model.

Table 1. Summary of the partial least squares (PLS) latent variable selection and model statistics for the off-line variables of glucose, VCD, lactate, and antibody concentration.

Off-Line Variable	Latent Variable Selection	Calibration (RMSE)	Validation (RMSEP)	Calibration (R^2)	Validation (R^2)
Glucose (g L^{-1})	7	0.19	0.38	0.97	0.88
VCD (1 × 10^6 cells mL^{-1})	7	1.78	3.49	0.99	0.96
Lactate (g L^{-1})	7	0.59	1.16	0.96	0.94
Antibody (g L^{-1})	7	0.17	0.09	0.99	0.94

Note: RMSE = root mean square error, RMSEP = root mean square error of prediction.

A comparison of the experimental recorded off-line variables to those predicted by the PLS models is shown in Figure 4. The PLS model for glucose concentration is shown to accurately predict the off-line measurements between the range of 1 and 5 g L^{-1}, as shown in Figure 4A. The RMSE and RMSEP of glucose concentration are equal to 0.19 and 0.38 g L^{-1}, respectively, which is equivalent to ±4.75% and ±9.5% of the glucose range investigated. Additionally, these values are below the typical measurement error of offline analysers of ~0.5 g L^{-1}. These predictions are comparable to the glucose predictions demonstrated by Rowland-Jones and Jaques [60], who observed an RMSE of 0.24 g L^{-1} and an RMSE of cross validation equal to 0.32 g L^{-1} using a similar type of Raman microscope during the at-line monitoring of a mammalian cell culture system in a miniature bioreactor system. The lactate predictions were slightly higher than those reported by Rowland-Jones and Jacques [60], who reported an RMSE of approximately 0.25 g L^{-1} and an RMSE cross validation of 0.30 g L^{-1}. However, the lactate predictions considered in this work were across a much wider concentration range, and demonstrate the ability of this tool to accurately predict lactate in excess of 12 g L^{-1}. The prediction accuracy of this HT-Raman microscope for both glucose and lactate is highly comparable to the on-line Raman spectroscopy sensors for mammalian cell culture systems reported in the approximate RMSEP range of 0.2–0.9 g L^{-1} for glucose concentration and 0.1–04 g L^{-1} for lactate [17,18,61]. The accuracy of these at-line predictions is comparable with the accuracy of the off-line nutrient analyser, and therefore has the potential to replace these analysers and help facilitate the development of an at-line glucose control strategy.

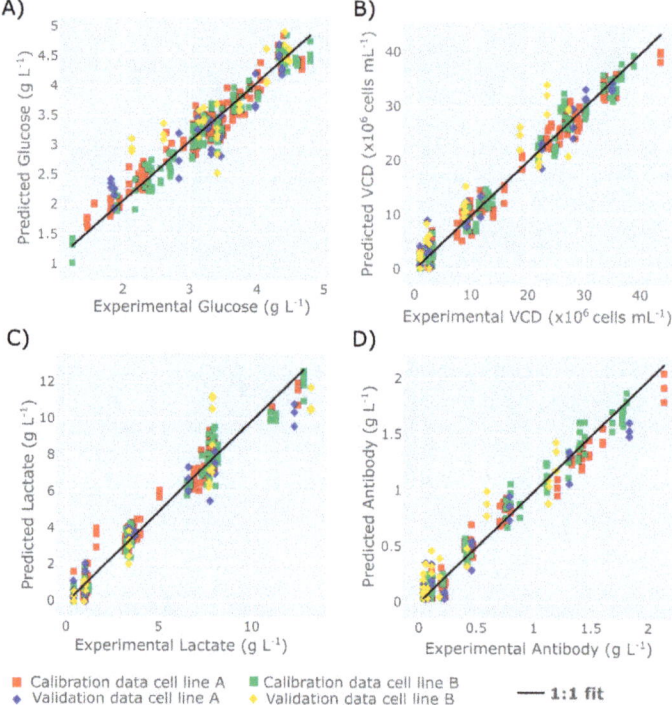

Figure 4. Parity plots demonstrating the prediction performance of four separate PLS models, highlighting the calibration and validation data sets of cell line A and B for (**A**) glucose concentration, (**B**) viable cell density (VCD), (**C**) lactate concentration, and (**D**) antibody concentration.

Four separate PLS models were built utilising 7 latent variables for each variable investigated, and calibrated using cell culture runs 1–5 and 7–11 from cell line A (indicated by the red squares) and runs 13–17 and 19–23 from cell line B (indicated by the green squares). The model was validated using cell culture runs 6 and 12 from cell line A (indicated by the blue diamonds) and runs 18 and 24 from cell line B (indicated by the yellow diamonds). The spectral data utilised in each PLS model were baseline-corrected spectra using a 1st order polynomial function, followed by the application of an SNV scattering scatter algorithm and a Savitzky–Golay smoothing filter.

Conventionally, the RMSE and RMSEP are the gold standard for model comparison and, provided the validation data set is independent, these metrics typically provide a good measure of the model's robustness. However, to further validate these model predictions the model coefficients should be scrutinised to ensure the model robustness, as outlined by the Raman spectroscopy model generation workflow defined in Figure 1. Within this work, the generated model was a PLS model, and the regression coefficients of the PLS model are shown in Figure 5. To assess whether the dominant wavenumbers highlighted by the PLS regression weights shown in Figure 5 are related to the variable of interest, a table containing the majority of the Raman vibrational peak assignments associated with each variable is shown in Table 2. This table highlights the associated Raman vibrational shifts expected after excitation from each variable due to changes in the molecular bond length such as stretching, which can be symmetric or asymmetric, or the bending of the molecular bond angles due to a wagging or a rocking motion. By comparing the expected Raman signature profile of these variables to the dominant peaks calculated by the PLS regression coefficients, the model's robustness can be evaluated. This ensures that the generated PLS model is specifically built to predict the variable investigated and not due to the metabolism-induced concentration correlations of other variables.

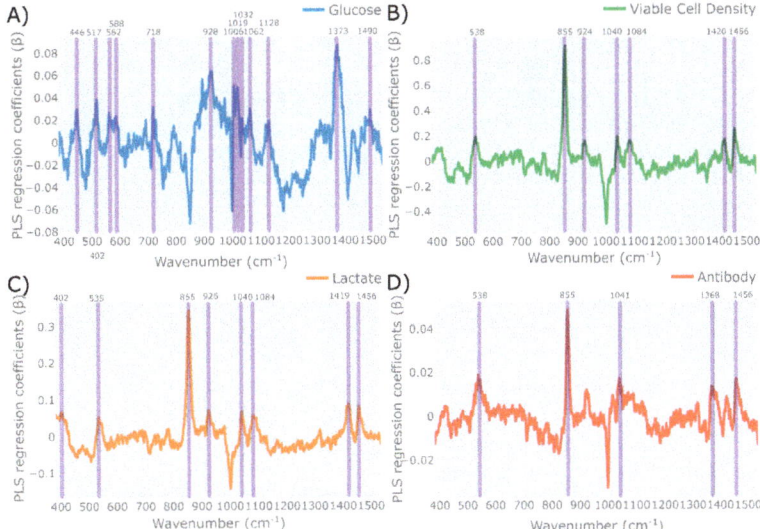

Figure 5. PLS regression coefficients (β) of each PLS model generated for (**A**) glucose, (**B**) viable cell density, (**C**) lactate, and (**D**) antibodies, with the wavenumbers corresponding to the Raman molecular signature of each variable highlighted by the shaded areas. The cut-off points for these PLS regression coefficients are glucose: $\beta > 0.02$; VCD: $\beta > 0.2$; lactate: $\beta > 0.05$; and antibody: $\beta > 0.015$. The spectral data utilised in each PLS model were baseline-corrected spectra using a 1st order polynomial function, followed by the application of an SNV scattering scatter algorithm and a Savitzky–Golay smoothing filter.

For glucose, the dominant regression coefficients were characterised by peaks that had a regression coefficient equal to or above 0.2 (i.e., $\beta > 0.02$). Wide peaks were characterised by the start, max, and end wavenumber of these peaks and by the max wavenumber value for narrow peaks. The majority of these peaks are shown to correctly align with the peaks associated with glucose, based on previously published literature defining the wavenumbers associated with glucose [62–68]. This includes the three distinct peaks in the 871–988 cm^{-1} range, which are indicated in Figure 5A as a single peak at wavenumber 928 cm^{-1}, which aligns with multiple literature references for the specific Raman scattering bands associated with glucose. The other dominant peaks at 1373, 1061, and 517 cm^{-1} all align with the expected peaks for glucose and further strengthen the predictions of the generated PLS model. Another interesting observation was outlined by Söderholm et al. [64], who demonstrated a small peak shift of approximate 2–5 wavenumbers depending on the glucose concentration in an aqueous solution with varying water contents; this demonstrates why, in Table 2, some of the regression peaks do not align precisely with those quoted in the literature. An additional evaluation of specific Raman bands for individual metabolites was defined by Singh et al. 2015 [65], who investigated the supernatants of a CHO cell culture grown in shake flasks using a Raman spectroscopy device. They used a classical least squares algorithm to determine, with a high degree of accuracy, the specific bands associated with both glucose and lactate. For glucose, they determined that there are seven characteristic peaks related to glucose, which are located at the wavelengths 435, 516, 990, 1076, 1121, 1374, and 1460 cm^{-1}, which all align with the dominant PLS regression coefficients features shown in Figure 5A. The alignment of these PLS regression coefficients with the expected Raman peaks of glucose provides additional confidence in this generated MVDA model. Similar observations were observed for the main regression peaks of lactate shown in Figure 5C that were highlighted for all the PLS regression coefficients above 0.05 (i.e., $\beta > 0.05$). The majority of these bands correspond to the Raman vibrational bands characterising lactate in the literature, as demonstrated in Table 2. Furthermore, Singh et al. characterised the main lactate-associated Raman peaks by wavenumbers 855, 922, 1045, 1085, and 1456 cm^{-1}, which align almost perfectly with those shown in Figure 5C. Similar to the glucose model, the correct alignment of the PLS regression coefficients with the expected lactate vibration bands provides the necessary confidence in the PLS model to enable subsequent predictions and deploy the MVDA model.

Figure 3B demonstrates the ability of this HT Raman spectroscopy to accurately predict the VCD across the expected range of mammalian cell cultures. The RMSEP for the VCD was 3.49×10^6 cells per mL^{-1}, which is equivalent to the ±9% measurement range investigated, and was found to accurately predict both high and low VCD concentrations for both cell lines, as shown in Figure 3B. The prediction accuracy is similar to that reported by Rowland-Jones et al., which was equal to 4.49×10^6 cells per mL^{-1}. These VCD predictions are also comparable to on-line Raman spectroscopy systems monitoring mammalian cell culture systems reporting predictions in the range of 1–5×10^6 cells per mL^{-1} [18,61]. The accuracy of these VCD measurements demonstrates the potential of this technology to replace the traditional off-line cell counter based on the accuracy of these predictions between the two cell lines investigated. However, as outlined in the Raman spectroscopy model generation workflow, it is necessary to evaluate the regression coefficients of the model.

The PLS regression coefficients of VCD are shown in Figure 5B, with the main peaks identified as those above 0.02 (i.e., $\beta > 0.02$), which are also indicated in Table 2. It is interesting to note that the primary peaks identified are also closely associated with the expected Raman vibrational bands of lactate. These highly correlated metabolite concentrations are problematic, as, although the RMSE and RMSEP of this PLS model are low, it is difficult to deconvolute this strong association with lactate. The correlation coefficient between the off-line lactate and off-line VCD concentrations was equal to 0.88, and therefore would help explain the location of these dominant lactate peaks corresponding to the calculated VCD regression coefficients. This is particularly evident when comparing the dominant lactate PLS regression peak shown at wavenumber 855 cm^{-1} in Figure 5C, which corresponds to the strong peak shown in the VCD at this precise wavenumber shown in Figure 5B. This high correlation is most likely due to the high accumulated lactate on days 6, 8, and 10, shown in Figure 2C, which resulted in a significant drop in the corresponding VCD values shown in Figure 2B. Based on a subsequent analysis of the PLS regression coefficients, it would be recommended to not deploy this PLS model for VCD and to generate additional experiment runs that do not result in a strong correlation between the off-line analytics of VCD and lactate.

The most promising application of this HT-Raman spectroscopy device is the ability to accurately predict the at-line product concentration, as shown in Figure 4D. The PLS model generated had an RMSE equal to 0.09 g L^{-1}, and the RMSEP was equal to 0.17 g L^{-1}, which is equivalent to ±4.5% and ±8.5% of the glucose range investigated. The accuracies of these predictions were similar to the RMSEP reported by Rowland-Jones et al. equal to 0.57 g L^{-1} [60], and slightly better than the RMSEP reported by on-line systems equal to 0.75–1.21 g L^{-1} [18]. The majority of previous research on Raman spectroscopy focuses on the nutrient concentration and cell concentrations, however the ability to measure product concentration opens up significant opportunities for the development of advanced control strategies. One demonstration was shown by Rowland-Jones and Jaques [60], who adapted nutrient and glucose feed additions through at-line predictions of glucose and VCD using a similar type of HT Raman spectroscopy microscope. This is one of the first demonstrations of PAT applied to control a miniature bioreactor system. The subsequent evaluation of the regression coefficients for the generated PLS model shown in Figure 5D highlights some issues with the robustness of this model. The dominant PLS regression coefficients for antibody were taken as those above 0.015 (i.e., $\beta > 0.015$). These peaks are shown to be primarily associated with either glucose or lactate. The strong lactate peak shown at wavenumber 855 cm^{-1} is evident from Figure 5D, and in addition to the strong glucose peak shown in Figure 5A at wavenumber 1373 cm^{-1} which can be observed at a similar location in the antibody wavenumber of 1368 cm^{-1}. Furthermore, the wavenumbers of 535, 1041, and 1456 cm^{-1} associated with lactate are also dominant for the PLS regression coefficients of the antibody. The strong association of antibody with both glucose and lactate can be partially explained by the high correlation coefficient (R^2) between the antibody and lactate equal to 0.77 and the antibody and glucose equal to −0.47. The issues with these metabolite-induced concentration correlations have been previously outlined by Rhiel et al. [69], who demonstrated that, due to the complex nature of the majority of bioprocesses, some analyte predictions using spectroscopic methods are based upon correlations between other variables. This was observed by Rheil et al. [69] during the analysis of the main metabolites of a CHO cell culture using a MIR probe. They demonstrated a similar strong independence between the majority of metabolite concentrations, which negatively affected their predictions. The strong correlation between the variables investigated in this research poses a major risk in subsequent predictions, where deviations in either glucose or lactate concentrations outside of the concentrations investigated in this work would drastically influence the antibody and VCD predictions. Subsequent experimental work is therefore needed to build more robust models that should include the spiking of these variables to build an independent data set to calibrate and validate these MVDA models.

Table 2. The dominant PLS regression peaks of glucose, lactate, VCD, and antibody and their corresponding Raman spectroscopy vibrational signatures based on previous literature values detailing reference wavenumbers for variables of interest.

Variable	PLS Regression Peak (β) Wavenumber [cm^{-1}] [USP Model]			Reference Wavenumber of Analyte [cm^{-1}]	Assignment	Reference
	start	max	end			

Table 2. Cont.

Variable	PLS Regression Peak (β) Wavenumber [cm⁻¹] [USP Model]			Reference Wavenumber of Analyte [cm⁻¹]	Assignment	Reference
Glucose *	442	446	450	443	-	[62]
				450	δ (C-C-O)	[63]
				451	-	[64]
	510	517	521	514	-	[62]
				516	-	[65]
				518	δ (C-CO)	[63]
	559	562	567	-	-	-
	583	588	590	585	δ (C-C-O)	[63]
	716	718	721	-	-	-
	871	928	988	893	ν (C-C)	[63]
				895	δ (C-H), δ (C-OH)	[66]
				898	-	[62]
				910	δ (C-H)	[63]
				913	-	[62]
				914	-	[67]
				990	-	[65]
		1006		1002	-	[67]
	1010	1019	1024	1018	δ (COH)	[68]
		1032		-	-	-
	1059	1062	1066	1060	ν (CO)	[63,66,68]
		1128		1120	δ (COH)	[63]
				1121	-	[65]
				1122	-	[67]
				1124	ν (CO)	[68]
				1125	ν (C-C)	[66]
				1130	-	[62]
	1358	1373	1395	1360	w (CH$_2$)	[63]
				1370	δ (C-H)	[66]
				1372	w (CH$_2$)	[68]
				1373	-	[62]
				1374	-	[65]
		1490		-	-	-
Lactate **	381	402	417	-	-	-
		535		540	w (CO$_2$-)	[70,71]
	840	855	866	855	-	[65]
				860	ν (C-CO$_2$-)	[70,71]
		926		930	r(CH$_3$)	[70,71]
		1040		1045	ν (C-CH$_3$)	[65,70,71]
		1084		1085	ν (C-O)	[65,70,71]
		1419		1420	ν (CO$_2$-)	[70,71]
		1456		1455	δ (CH$_3$)	[70,71]
				1456	-	[65]
VCD ***		538		540	lactate (w (CO$_2$-))	[70,71]
	840	855	866	855	-	[65]
				860	lactate ν (C-CO$_2$-)	[70,71]
		924		930	lactate (r (CH$_3$))	[70,71]
		1040		1045	lactate (ν (C-CH$_3$))	[65,70,71]
		1084		1085	lactate (ν (C-O))	[65,70,71]
		1420		1420	lactate (ν (CO$_2$-))	[70,71]
		1456		1455	lactate (δ (CH$_3$))	[70,71]
				1456	-	[65]

Table 2. Cont.

Variable	PLS Regression Peak (β) Wavenumber [cm⁻¹] [USP Model]			Reference Wavenumber of Analyte [cm⁻¹]	Assignment	Reference
Antibody ****			538	540	lactate (w (CO$_2$-))	[70,71]
	843	855	864	855	-	[65]
				860	lactate ν (C-CO2-)	[70,71]
		1041		1045	lactate (ν (C-CH$_3$))	[65,70,71]
				1360	glucose (w (CH$_2$))	[63]
	1362	1368	1384	1370	glucose (δ (C-H))	[66]
				1372	glucose (w (CH$_2$))	[68]
				1373	-	[62]
				1374	-	[65]
	1453	1456	1466	1455	lactate (δ (CH$_3$))	[70,71]
				1456	-	[65]

Note: w = wagging, δ = bending, ν = stretching, r = rocking. Cut-off points for PLS regression coefficient are glucose: * β > 0.02; lactate: ** β > 0.05; VCD *** β > 0.2; antibody **** β > 0.15.

This ability to monitor these CPPs through at-line measurements opens up additional opportunities for the development of advanced control strategies for miniature bioreactor systems. The reduction in the necessary sample volume could enable more frequent at-line sampling, such as every 6 or 12 h, enhancing the monitoring and control of these miniature bioreactor systems. The application of advanced control strategies earlier in the process development cycle encourages the integration of PAT within future scale-up and commercial operations.

3.2. Application of Raman Spectroscopy to DSP

In this study, an HT InVia Raman Microscope was used to determine the total concentration and monomer purity of Fc-fusion protein during CEX chromatography purification in order to guide sample prioritisation for further analytical methods, such as the HPLC-SEC-based determination of monomer purity and UV absorbance at 280 nm for the total protein concentration.

The data set was based on a total of 18 individual CEX runs, including both step and gradient elution, resulting in total of 201 individual elution fraction samples, each of which were measured in duplicate, producing a total of 402 spectra. Only elution fractions above 0.5 mg/mL were included in the data set (as measured off-line by A280), as that was the previously estimated sensitivity of the device.

The PLS models were built as described in Section 2.9, and followed the Raman spectroscopy model generation workflow defined in Figure 1. The number of latent variables for the PLS model were based on minimising the RMSE and RMSEP. The validation and calibration sets showed a range of elution buffer conditions, where the PLS calibration set consisted of elution fractions from runs using 20 mM of sodium citrate, with varying levels of sodium chloride (0–0.5 M). There were two district validation sets—the first (P1) was in the identical buffer range as the calibration set and consisted of 40 samples, whereas the second (P2) consisted of elution fractions using elution buffer containing 50 mM of sodium citrate, as well as wider salt range (133–210 mM), and consisted of 22 samples. The product concentrations in the data sets ranged from 0.5 to 33.1 mg/mL for T1, 0.7 to 19.41 mg/mL for P1, and 1.7 to 33.2 mg/mL for P2. The monomer purity ranged from to 70% to 100% for all three data sets, with up to 20% HMW species and up to 20% LMW species. These two data sets were chosen in order to test the robustness of the model to changes in salt concentrations and sample matrices typically seen in purification processes.

The PLS model describing product concentration is shown in Figure 6. Using seven LVs, the model has resulted in an excellent degree of fit (Table 3), with an R^2 (T1) = 0.99 for the calibration sample set (4A) and R^2 (P1) = 0.99 and R^2 (P2) = 0.98 for the validation sets P1 (4B) and P2 (4C), respectively. The RMSEP of 1.09 mg/mL for P1 and 3.54 for P2 corresponds to 6.1% and 11.2% of the range. A higher error for validation set P2 is expected, due to wider range of buffer conditions relative to the calibration set.

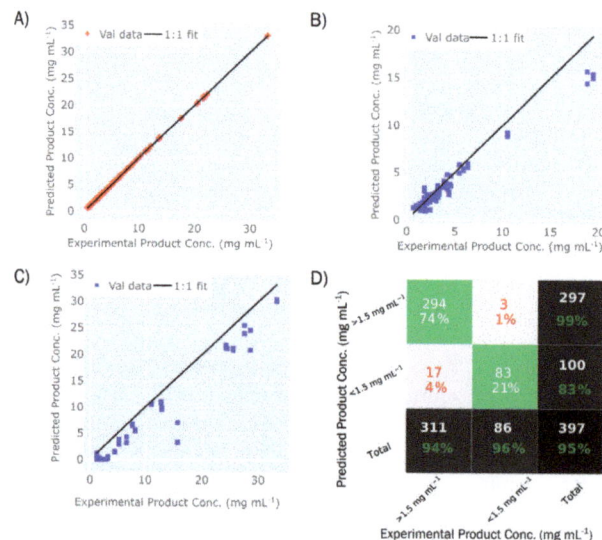

Figure 6. Prediction performance of the PLS model predicting product concentration with (**A**) displaying a parity plot for validation set T1, (**B**) parity plot for calibration set P1, (**C**) parity plot for calibration set P2, and (**D**) confusion matrix that classifies the product concentration predictions above or below 1.5 g L^{-1} in comparison to the experimental product concentrations. In the confusion matrix (**D**), the top left cell indicates true positives, the top middle cell indicates false positives, the middle left cell indicates false negatives, and the middle cell indicates true negatives. In each of these matrix cells, the value indicates the number and percentage of samples in each category. In the total matrix cell columns and rows, the total number of samples is given, with the percentage indicating the number of true positives or true negatives.

Table 3. Summary of monomer purity and product concentration model fit (R^2), RMSE of calibration set, and RMSEP of two validation sets.

Statistical Measure of Fit	Calibration (T1)	Validation (P1)	Validation (P2)
	Product concentration (mg mL^{-1})		
R^2	0.99	0.99	0.98
RMSE/RMSEP	0.16	1.09	3.62
	Monomer concentration (%)		
R^2	0.98	0.86	0.34
RMSE/RMSEP	1.09	4.27	13.68

Note: RMSE = root mean square error (used for calibration), RMSEP = root mean square error of prediction (used for validation).

Furthermore, the model was used to classify samples based on whether or not the concentrations were higher than 1.5 mg/mL (Figure 6D). This value of 1.5 mg/mL was selected as the cut-off point to determine low-concentration samples; any samples below this concentration limit would not be further analysed by high-performance liquid chromatography (HPLC). Since only samples above 0.5 mg/mL were included in the spectral measurements, the classification was working within a narrow range of 0.5 and 1.5 mg/mL. Within this range, 95% of samples were classified correctly, of which 74% were true positives (concentration above 1.5 mg/mL) and 21% were true negatives (concentration below 1.5 mg/mL). The classification model classified both samples that were not part of the training set (P1 and P2), as well as samples that were used to build the model (T1), which leads to the accuracy of prediction being higher than what would be seen if only previously unknown samples were used. Nevertheless, this shows that the model can be used to determine which samples should be considered for further analysis and pooling, and which can be discarded at this stage due to no or low levels of protein.

The second variable of interest was monomer purity, as it is desirable to achieve maximal monomer purity whilst minimising the presence of aggregated (HMW) or fragmented (LMW) species, or both. In this experiment, a model was built that predicted monomer purity (Figure 5), although with a relatively large RMSE, which would not allow for quantitative detection, but could serve to distinguish between samples with high purity versus samples with low purity, and therefore save time for more laborious methods such as HPLC.

The model predicting monomer purity was based on the same data set as the total concentration model, with the exception that only samples with concentrations above 1.5 mg/mL were used. The model uses eight LVs. The summary of model statistics is shown in Table 3. The PLS calibration model for monomer purity resulted in an R^2 (T1) = 0.98 (5A), R^2 (P1) = 0.86 (5B), and R^2 (P2) = 0.34 (7C), as shown in Figure 7. The RMSEP for monomer purity for P1 and P2 corresponds to 4.27% and 13.68%, respectively. The model was further used to classify samples according to a monomer purity of 90% or higher, where a total of 92% of the samples were classified correctly as either true positives (80%) or true negatives (13%), as is shown in Figure 7D.

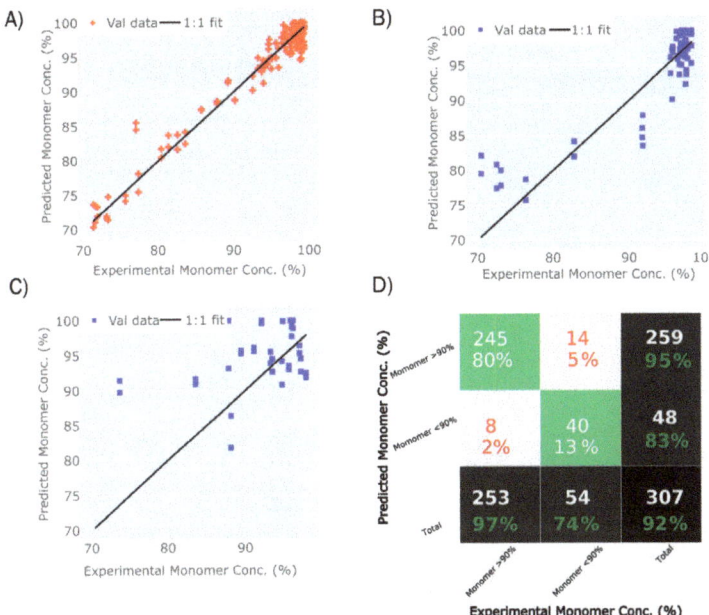

Figure 7. Prediction performance of the PLS model predicting the monomer purity of the fusion protein with (**A**) displaying a parity plot for validation set T1, (**B**) parity plot for calibration set P1, (**C**) parity plot for calibration set P2, and (**D**) confusion matrix that classifies the monomer purity predictions above or below 90% in comparison to the experimental monomer purity.

In the confusion matrix (**D**), the top left cell indicates true positives, the top middle cell indicates false positives, the middle left cell indicates false negatives, and the middle cell indicates true negatives. In each of these matrix cells, the value indicates the number and percentage of samples in each category. In the total matrix cell columns and rows, the total number of samples is given, with the percentage indicating the number of true positives or true negatives.

When validated using the two prediction sets, a relatively low RMSEP was achieved for data set P1, and no useful predictions were achieved for set P2. This led us to believe that the model was based on features that are absent from the P2 data set, which might be caused by changes in the elution profile and the content of co-eluting impurities. Alternatively, the type of HMW/LMW species might differ between data sets P1 and P2 due to changes in the elution buffer. Despite that, the model is capable of classifying samples with an acceptable degree of accuracy.

The PLS model developed for product concentration was found to have a significantly lower RMSEP, and was less susceptible to changes in the sample matrix conditions than the PLS for monomer purity. Examining the PLS regression plots for the concentration model (described in Table 4 and Figure 8A), multiple IgG spectral features can be identified, such as the Amide I and Amide III bands at wavelengths 1673 cm^{-1}, and 1236 and 1337 cm^{-1}, respectively. Bands resulting from the vibrations of amino acid groups can be further found at 757 and 1553 cm^{-1} for tryptophan, 1003 and 1208 cm^{-1} for phenylalanine, and 1208 cm^{-1} for tyrosine [72–74]. Regression coefficients corresponding to the IgG peaks as annotated in the literature suggest that the model is valid and is based directly on the protein spectra rather than on the spectral features of other correlated components.

Table 4. PLS dominant regression peaks of protein and IgG aggregates associated with monomer and product concentrations and their corresponding Raman spectroscopy vibrational signatures, based on previous literature values detailing reference wavenumbers for the variables of interest.

Variable	PLS Regression Peak (β) Wavenumber [cm^{-1}] [DSP Model]			Reference Wavenumber of Analyte [cm^{-1}]	Assignment	Reference
	start	max	end			
Protein **** (Fc-fusion *****)		757		758 759	Trp	[72] [73]
		1003		1002 1004 1005	Phe	[74] [72] [73]
		1029		-	-	-
		1208		1210	Tyr; Phe	
		1236		1239 1243	Amide III	[74] [72]
		1337		1340	Amide III	[73]
		1447		1450 1451	CH2 def	[73] [72]
		1553		1552 1554	Trp	[72] [73]
		1673		1673	Amide I	[74]
Protein aggregate	831	863	901	830; 850 878	Tyr Tyr	[45] [73]
	1437	1448	1446	-	Tyr Tyr	[45] [73]

Note: Trp = Tryptophan, Tyr = Tyrosine, Phe = Phenylalanine. **** Cut-off points for PLS regression coefficients product β > 0.0025; monomer β > 0.05. ***** Approximate assignment, as reference peaks correspond to human IgG, whereas the investigated protein is an Fc-fusion protein.

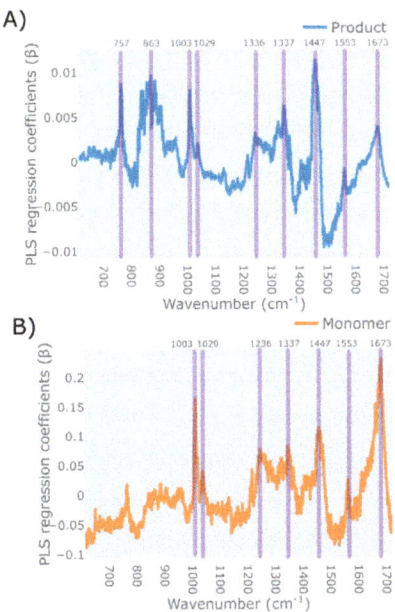

Figure 8. PLS regression coefficient (β) plots for each PLS model generated for (**A**) the monomer purity model and (**B**) product concentration, with the wavenumbers corresponding to the Raman molecular signature of each variable highlighted by the shaded areas. The cut-off points for these PLS regression coefficients are product: β > 0.005; monomer β > 0.075. The PLS model for monomer purity was developed using the raw spectra. The PLS model for the product concentration was developed using spectra that was baseline-corrected using a 1st order polynomial function, followed by the application of an SNV scattering scatter algorithm and a Savitzky–Golay smoothing filter. The PLS model for product concentration utilised 7 latent variables and the model for monomer purity utilised 8 latent variables.

The PLS regression plot for monomer purity in Figure 8A relies on the above-mentioned general protein peaks, as can be seen based on the similarities between the two plots, but also has additional features, especially in the area between wavelengths 831–901 cm^{-1} and 1437–1446 cm^{-1}. Neither of the two regions correspond to the spectrum of the citrate buffer (data not shown). Although difficult to determine without further experimental data, this might correspond to aggregation, as the wavelength region has previously been suggested to correspond to a shift in the tyrosine Fermi doublet at 830/850, which is seem upon aggregation [45].

The results show that HT-Raman spectroscopy has the potential to support downstream development through the rapid determination of product concentration and monomer purity, which enables the prioritisation of samples for further analysis and therefore saves operator and instrument time. We have shown that robust product predictions can be achieved, in line with the previously published literature, but predictions of monomer concentrations had a relatively large RMSEP and lower robustness. In order to make the Raman spectroscopy truly attractive to DSP, improvements in terms of sensitivity need to be made.

Studies have described various spectral changes upon protein aggregation [45,46], although the spectral features do not seem to be very consistent and might differ from product to product. As a consequence, the PLS model described here might be relying on a combination of background signal peaks and concentration peaks, rather than the specific spectral signal for aggregation and/or fragmentation. This would also explain why the model predictions are significantly worse for the P2 data set, where the elution buffer was changed, which likely results in changes to the background spectra due to the changed sample matrix.

A specific spectral signature for aggregation/fragmentation might potentially be present, but the sensitivity of the set-up could be insufficient to detect it. The majority of samples had a relatively low aggregate content (below 5%), which would result in aggregate concentrations of about 0.025 to 1.655 mg/mL. Based on previous experiments, we have estimated the LOD at around 1 mg/mL; hence, a large portion of the aggregate content in the samples might be below the limit. We have shown ways to increase the sensitivity, including a change in the 96-well plate material, laser output, and objective magnification, which would likely increase the sensitivity of the model.

Although a reduction in number of samples for HPLC analysis might be welcomed by the operators of such instruments, it might not necessarily justify the acquisition of such equipment. The major simplification of large screening experiments could be enabled by the ability to predict robustly monomer purity, especially in situations where LMW/HMW species elute throughout the main monomer peak without clear separation. The ultimate application of the technology would be the real-time detection of multiple CQAs based on the Raman spectra, potentially integrated with currently monitored variables such as UV, pH, osmolarity, etc. This would allow real-time control, leading to a higher product quality and ultimately supporting initiatives such as continuous manufacturing. This work is the first step towards such applications, as it highlights the current limitations as well as the potential improvements that can be implemented.

3.2.1. Strategies for Improving Predictions

Considering the high RMSEP of the monomer purity model, efforts were made to increase the sensitivity of the instrument by the optimisation of the acquisition settings. Adjustments to the acquisition settings were made to improve the signal intensity, including a change in the sample holder, microscope objective, and laser power. The data presented in this study were acquired using polypropylene 96-well plates, which were switched to stainless steel in order to improve the signal. As shown in Figure 9, there is a significant reduction in background between the PP plates and the steel plates. Furthermore, when the acquisition was performed using a 50X long-working distance objective, the background signal was further decreased, especially in the spectral range of the water peak (1300–1500 cm^{-1}). Additional improvement in the spectral quality came from using the higher laser power (300 mW vs. 30 mW), which was enabled through the switch to steel plates, as using a high laser power in the polypropylene plates caused the scorching of the plate and heating of the sample.

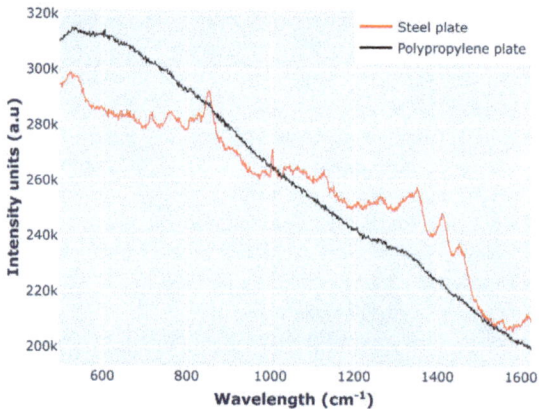

Figure 9. Comparison of acquisition settings of the spectra recorded by HT Raman spectroscopy microscope using polypropylene plates (in black) compared to the improved acquisition settings using stainless steel (SS) plates, a higher laser power, and higher magnification objective (in red).

3.2.2. Raman Spectroscopy Future Perspective

Raman spectroscopy has positioned itself as the leading on-line and at-line process analyser for biopharmaceutical processes. This technology is non-invasive, non-destructive, and has little interference with water, making it an ideal tool for both USP and DSP operations. One of the primary challenges of Raman spectroscopy is the weak Raman signal that reduces the sensitivity of the instrument and can be further hindered by background fluorescence, which, as demonstrated in this work, is highly problematic during the analysis of biological samples. Pre-processing the spectra can alleviate the majority of this fluorescence and ensure that accurate MVDA models can be generated to predict the variable of interest. However, ensuring the developed MVDA model predictions have a low RMSE and low RMSEP does not always guarantee a robust accurate model. To ensure the developed MVDA model is sufficient, an in-depth evaluation of the regression weights is required. In order to build a robust MVDA model, the regression coefficients should correspond to the correct wavenumbers associated with the specific molecular vibration bonds associated with the Raman scattering of the variable. This work provides two useful tables (Tables 2 and 4) outlining some of the primary vibrational modes related to Raman scattering associated with glucose, lactate, and protein based upon the previously published literature. This work demonstrated that, although the PLS model generated for the antibody and VCD concentrations resulted in a low RMSE and RMSEP, the regression weights of these models did not correspond to the antibody and VCD molecular vibrations; instead, they corresponded to only those wavenumbers associated with lactate and glucose molecular vibrations. Therefore, these metabolism-induced concentration correlations could lead to poor VCD and antibody predictions when either the glucose or lactate concentrations differed from the current glucose and lactate concentrations in this experiment. Therefore, the Raman spectroscopy model generation workflow outlined in Figure 1 highlights the importance of analysing the MVDA regression coefficients to ensure they align with the expected vibrational bonds associated with the variable, in addition to presenting the traditional RMSE and RMSEP metrics. This paper also demonstrates the value of an HT Raman spectroscopy device and its potential to revolutionise the monitoring and control of automated microbioreactor systems. Although improvements to the prediction accuracy of the models are needed, HT Raman spectroscopy has the potential to replace the need for additional analytic equipment, which can reduce operating costs. The additional benefit of the HT-Raman spectroscopy device is its ability to analyse samples across both USP and DSP operations.

4. Conclusions

This paper demonstrates the value of implementing MVDA to complex spectral data sets generated by an HT-Raman spectroscopy microscope to support the at-line monitoring and subsequent optimisation of USP and DSP operations, particularly those activities in early-stage development with limited sample volume availability. The USP case study investigated the ability of this device to predict the key process parameters typically measured off-line during cell culture for two different cell lines grown in a micro-bioreactor system cultivating 24 cell culture runs. The Raman spectra recorded throughout this mammalian cell culture was analysed using the Raman spectroscopy model generation workflow outlined in this paper and enabled the development of an optimised PLS model resulting in accurate predictions of the glucose, lactate, viable cell density, and product concentration. The RMSE and RMSEP were comparable to previously reported in-line Raman spectroscopy probes. However, upon the investigation of the regression coefficients of these variables, the VCD and antibody PLS models were shown to be primarily correlated with the Raman vibrational signatures of lactate and glucose. Therefore, subsequent experimentation is required to validate the robustness of these models. However, these results demonstrate the potential of this technology to predict these off-line variables using a single analytic device in comparison to three separate off-line analysers, which could greatly simplify the monitoring of these micro-bioreactor systems. Additionally, these at-line measurements require less volume than traditional analytic methods. This opens up opportunities for advanced control strategies and helps promote the inclusion of PAT in early-stage process development, thus simplifying the adoption of PAT within commercial-scale manufacturing.

The second case study involved a commercial DSP unit operation and further demonstrates the versatility and flexibility of this instrument. This case study focused on streamlining the sample collection of the CEX chromatography step, investigating different elution conditions during the purification of a fusion protein. The HT Raman microscope collected spectral data on 18 CEX runs operated in both step and gradient elution modes; these runs were operated using different buffer conditions. The potential of the Raman spectra to predict the total protein concentration and monomer purity was investigated. Both variables were modelled by an optimised PLS model leveraging the data from the Raman spectra. To demonstrate the robustness of the developed PLS model, two distinct validation data sets were considered. The first calibration data set (P1) included identical buffers that were in the same range as those used to calibrate the model. The second calibration data (P2) contained elution fractions that used a buffer containing 50 mM of sodium citrate and a wider salt range that was outside of the ranges of the validation data set. It was shown that the use of HT-Raman enables relatively accurate predictions of the protein concentration and monomer purity, however when the model was validated using a sample set with a different buffer background (P2), a significant decrease in prediction accuracy was observed, suggesting separate models might have to be built for specific conditions.

In summary, the HT-Raman spectroscopy microscope demonstrated significant potential as a novel cross-functional PAT applicable to both USP and DSP operations. The device was shown to accurately predict the primary CPPs in USP and the CQAs relevant to DSP through the application of MVDA. Furthermore, this technology has the potential to reduce the reliance on multiple separate analytic devices, thus reducing the capital and operating costs. Additionally, the near real-time information generated can be further exploited to develop and implement advanced control strategies and process optimisation earlier in the process development lifecycle.

Author Contributions: A.U. and S.G. contributed equally to this work. Conceptualisation, S.G., A.U., A.T., M.C., R.T., A.C., M.H., C.S., and S.S.F.; methodology, S.G., A.U., A.T., A.C., K.L., R.Z., M.H., and C.S.; software, A.U., S.G., and C.S.; validation, S.G., A.U., and C.S.; formal analysis, A.U., A.T., R.Z., A.C., K.L., S.G., and C.S.; investigation, S.G., A.U., A.T., A.C., R.Z., K.L., M.H., and C.S.; resources, M.C., R.T., A.C., M.H., and S.S.F.; data curation, A.U., K.L., R.Z., S.G., and C.P.; writing—original draft preparation, S.G., A.U., and C.S.; writing—review and editing, A.U., S.G., A.T., M.C., C.S., and S.S.F.; visualisation, S.G. and A.U.; supervision, M.C., R.T., A.C., C.S., M.H., and S.S.F.; funding acquisition, R.T., M.C., A.C., M.H., and S.S.F. All authors have read and agreed to the published version of the manuscript.

Funding: This research is associated with the joint UCL-AstraZeneca Centre of Excellence for predictive multivariate decision support tools in the bioprocessing sector, and financial support for S.G. and R.Z is gratefully acknowledged. Furthermore, support from EPSRC for S.G. is also greatly appreciated (EP/I033270/1). UCL Biochemical Engineering hosts the Future Targeted Healthcare Manufacturing Hub (Grant Reference: EP/P006485/1) in collaboration with UK universities and with funding from the UK Engineering and Physical Sciences Research Council (EPSRC) and a consortium of industrial users and sector organisations.

Conflicts of Interest: The authors declare no conflict of interest.

Abbreviations

AUC	Area under curve
CEX	Cation exchange chromatography
CHO	Chinese hamster ovary
CPP	Critical process parameters
CQA	Critical quality attribute
DLS	Dynamic light scattering
DSP	Downstream processing

FDA	Food and drug administration
GMP	Good manufacturing practice
HCP	Host cell proteins
HMW	High molecular weight
HPLC	High performance liquid chromatography
HT	High throughput
IEX	Ion exchange
LMW	Low molecular Weight
MIR	Mid-infrared
MVDA	Multivariate data analysis
NIR	Near-infrared
PAT	Process analytical technology
PLS	Partial least squares
PLS-DA	Partial least squares discrimination analysis
RMSE	Root mean square error
RMSEP	Root mean square error of prediction
R^2	Correlation coefficient
R&D	Research and development
SE	Size exclusion
SERS	Surface-enhanced Raman Spectroscopy
SNV	Standard normal variate
SS	Stainless steel
UHPLC	Ultra high-performance liquid chromatography
USP	Upstream processing
UV	Ultraviolet
VCD	Viable cell density

References

1. PAT—A Framework for Innovative Pharmaceutical, Manufacturing and Quality Assurance. Available online: https://www.fda.gov/media/71012/download (accessed on 1 September 2020).
2. Brunner, M.; Fricke, J.; Kroll, P.; Herwig, C. Investigation of the interactions of critical scale-up parameters (pH, pO_2 and pCO_2) on CHO batch performance and critical quality attributes. *Bioprocess Biosyst. Eng.* **2017**, *40*, 251–263. [CrossRef] [PubMed]
3. Rathore, A.S.; Kapoor, G. Process analytical technology: Strategies for biopharmaceuticals. In *Encyclopedia of Industrial Biotechnology: Bioprocess, Bioseparation, and Cell Technology*; Flickinger, M., Ed.; John Wiley & Sons: Hoboken, NJ, USA, 2010; pp. 1543–1565.
4. Biophorum. In-Line Monitoring/Real-Time Release Testing in Biopharmaceutical Processes—Prioritization and Cost Benefit Analysis. Available online: https://www.biophorum.com/download/in-line-monitoring-real-time-release-testing-in-biopharmaceutical-processes-prioritization-and-cost-benefit-analysis (accessed on 1 September 2020).
5. Challa, S.; Potumarthi, R. Chemometrics-based process analytical technology (PAT) tools: Applications and adaptation in pharmaceutical and biopharmaceutical industries. *Appl. Biochem. Biotechnol.* **2013**, *169*, 66–76. [CrossRef] [PubMed]
6. Konakovsky, V.; Yagtu, A.C.; Clemens, C.; Müller, M.M.; Berger, M.; Schlatter, S.; Herwig, C. Universal capacitance model for real-time biomass in cell culture. *Sensors* **2015**, *15*, 22128–22150. [CrossRef] [PubMed]
7. Hakemeyer, C.; Strauss, U.; Werz, S.; Jose, G.E.; Folque, F.; Menezes, J.C. At-line NIR spectroscopy as effective PAT monitoring technique in Mab cultivations during process development and manufacturing. *Talanta* **2012**, *90*, 12–21. [CrossRef] [PubMed]
8. Sandor, M.; Rüdinger, F.; Bienert, R.; Grimm, C.; Solle, D.; Scheper, T. Comparative study of non-invasive monitoring via infrared spectroscopy for mammalian cell cultivations. *J. Biotechnol.* **2013**, *168*, 636–645. [CrossRef] [PubMed]

9. Ude, C.; Schmidt-Hager, J.; Findeis, M.; John, G.T.; Scheper, T.; Beutel, S. Application of an online-biomass sensor in an optical multisensory platform prototype for growth monitoring of biotechnical relevant microorganism and cell lines in single-use shake flasks. *Sensors* **2014**, *14*, 17390–17405. [CrossRef]
10. Ude, C.; Schmidt-Hager, J.; Findeis, M.; John, G.T.; Scheper, T.; Beutel, S. Fluorescence-based soft sensor for at situ monitoring of chinese hamster ovary cell cultures. *Biotechnol. Bioeng.* **2014**, *111*, 1577–1586.
11. Calvet, A.; Li, B.; Ryder, A.G. Rapid quantification of tryptophan and tyrosine in chemically defined cell culture media using fluorescence spectroscopy. *J. Pharm. Biomed. Anal.* **2012**, *71*, 89–98. [CrossRef]
12. Goldrick, S.; Lovett, D.; Montague, G.; Lennox, B. Influence of Incident Wavelength and Detector Material Selection on Fluorescence in the Application of Raman Spectroscopy to a Fungal Fermentation Process. *Bioengineering* **2018**, *5*, 79. [CrossRef]
13. Buckley, K.; Ryder, A.G. Applications of Raman Spectroscopy in Biopharmaceutical Manufacturing: A Short Review. *Appl. Spectrosc.* **2017**, *71*, 1085–1116. [CrossRef]
14. Wu, Q.; Hamilton, T.; Nelson, W.H.; Elliott, S.; Sperry, J.F.; Wu, M. UV Raman Spectral Intensities of E. Coli and Other Bacteria Excited at 228.9, 244.0, and 248.2 nm. *Anal. Chem.* **2001**, *73*, 3432–3440. [CrossRef] [PubMed]
15. Matthews, T.E.; Berry, B.N.; Smelko, J.; Moretto, J.; Moore, B.; Wiltberger, K. Closed loop control of lactate concentration in mammalian cell culture by Raman spectroscopy leads to improved cell density, viability, and biopharmaceutical protein production. *Biotechnol. Bioeng.* **2016**, *113*, 2416–2424. [CrossRef] [PubMed]
16. Matthews, T.E.; Smelko, J.P.; Berry, B.; Romero-Torres, S.; Hill, D.; Kshirsagar, R.; Wiltberger, K. Glucose monitoring and adaptive feeding of mammalian cell culture in the presence of strong autofluorescence by near infrared Raman spectroscopy. *Biotechnol. Prog.* **2018**, *34*, 1574–1580. [CrossRef] [PubMed]
17. Abu-Absi, N.R.; Kenty, B.M.; Cuellar, M.E.; Borys, M.C.; Sakhamuri, S.; Strachan, D.J.; Hausladen, M.C.; Li, Z.J. Real time monitoring of multiple parameters in mammalian cell culture bioreactors using an in-line Raman spectroscopy probe. *Biotechnol. Bioeng.* **2011**, *108*, 1215–1221. [CrossRef]
18. Webster, T.A.; Hadley, B.C.; Hilliard, W.; Jaques, C.; Mason, C. Development of generic raman models for a GS-KOTM CHO platform process. *Biotechnol. Prog.* **2018**, *34*, 730–737. [CrossRef]
19. Craven, S.J.; Whelan, J.; Glennon, B. Glucose concentration control of a fed-batch mammalian cell bioprocess using a nonlinear model predictive controller. *J. Process Control* **2014**, *24*, 344–357. [CrossRef]
20. Rafferty, C.; O'Mahony, J.; Burgoyne, B.; Rea, R.; Balss, K.M.; Latshaw, D.C. Raman spectroscopy as a method to replace off-line pH during mammalian cell culture processes. *Biotechnol. Bioeng.* **2020**, *117*, 146–156. [CrossRef]
21. Li, M.Y.; Ebel, B.; Blanchard, F.; Paris, C.; Guedon, E.; Marc, A. Control of IgG glycosylation by in situ and real-time estimation of specific growth rate of CHO cells cultured in bioreactor. *Biotechnol. Bioeng.* **2019**, *116*, 985–993. [CrossRef]
22. Hong, P.; Koza, S.; Bouvier, E.S.P. A review size exclusion chromatography for the analysis of protein biotherapeutics and their aggregates. *J. Liq. Chromatogr. Relat. Technol.* **2012**, *35*, 2923–2950. [CrossRef]
23. Fekete, S.; Beck, A.; Veuthey, J.L.; Guillarme, D. Theory and practice of size exclusion chromatography for the analysis of protein aggregates. *J. Pharm. Biomed. Anal.* **2014**, *101*, 161–173. [CrossRef]
24. Swartz, M.E. UPLC™: An Introduction and Review. *J. Liq. Chromatogr. Relat. Technol.* **2005**, *28*, 1253–1263. [CrossRef]
25. Bouvier, E.S.P.; Koza, S.M. Advances in size-exclusion separations of proteins and polymers by UHPLC. *TrAC Trends Anal. Chem.* **2014**, *63*, 85–94. [CrossRef]
26. Haberger, M.; Leiss, M.; Heidenreich, A.K.; Pester, O.; Hafenmair, G.; Hook, M.; Bonnington, L.; Wegele, H.; Haindl, M.; Reusch, D.; et al. Rapid characterization of biotherapeutic proteins by size-exclusion chromatography coupled to native mass spectrometry. *mAbs* **2016**, *8*, 331–339. [CrossRef] [PubMed]
27. Madadkar, P.; Umatheva, U.; Hale, G.; Durocher, Y.; Ghosh, R. Ultrafast Separation and Analysis of Monoclonal Antibody Aggregates Using Membrane Chromatography. *Anal. Chem.* **2017**, *89*, 4716–4720. [CrossRef]
28. Tiwari, A.; Kateja, N.; Chanana, S.; Rathore, A.S. Use of HPLC as an Enabler of Process Analytical Technology in Process Chromatography. *Anal. Chem.* **2018**, *90*, 7824–7829. [CrossRef]

29. Patel, B.A.; Pinto, N.D.; Gospodarek, A.; Kilgore, B.; Goswami, K.; Napoli, W.N.; Desai, J.; Heo, J.H.; Panzera, D.; Pollard, D.; et al. On-Line Ion Exchange Liquid Chromatography as a Process Analytical Technology for Monoclonal Antibody Characterization in Continuous Bioprocessing. *Anal. Chem.* **2017**, *89*, 11357–11365. [CrossRef]
30. Heo, J.H.; Heo, J.H.; Mou, X.; Wang, F.; Troisi, J.M.; Christopher, W.S.; Kirby, S.; Driscoll, D.; Mercorelli, S.; Pollard, D.J. A microfluidic approach to high throughput quantification of host cell protein impurities for bioprocess development. *Pharm. Bioprocess.* **2014**, *2*, 129–139. [CrossRef]
31. Kumar, M.A.; Mazlomi, M.A.; Hedström, M.; Mattiasson, B. Versatile automated continuous flow system (VersAFlo) for bioanalysis and bioprocess control. *Sens. Actuators B Chem.* **2012**, *161*, 855–861. [CrossRef]
32. Rüdt, M.; Briskot, T.; Hubbuch, J. Advances in downstream processing of biologics—Spectroscopy: An emerging process analytical technology. *J. Chromatogr. A* **2017**, *1490*, 2–9. [CrossRef]
33. Rolinger, L.; Rüdt, M.; Hubbuch, J. A critical review of recent trends, and a future perspective of optical spectroscopy as PAT in biopharmaceutical downstream processing. *Anal. Bioanal. Chem.* **2020**, *412*, 2047–2064. [CrossRef]
34. Rüdt, M.; Brestrich, N.; Rolinger, L.; Hubbuch, J. Real-time monitoring and control of the load phase of a protein a capture step. *Biotechno. Bioeng.* **2017**, *114*, 368–373. [CrossRef] [PubMed]
35. Brestrich, N.; Ruedt, M.; Buechler, D.; Hubbuch, J. Selective protein quantification for preparative chromatography using variable pathlength UV/Vis spectroscopy and partial least squares regression. *Chem. Eng. Sci.* **2018**, *176*, 157–164. [CrossRef]
36. Rolinger, L.; Ruedt, M.; Diehm, J.; Chow-Hubbertz, J.; Heitmann, M.; Schleper, S.; Hubbuch, J. Multi-attribute PAT for UF/DF of Proteins—Monitoring Concentration, particle sizes, and Buffer Exchange. *Anal. Bioanal. Chem.* **2020**, *412*, 2123–2136. [CrossRef]
37. Thakur, G.; Hebbi, V.; Rathore, A.S. An NIR-based PAT approach for real-time control of loading in Protein a chromatography in continuous manufacturing of monoclonal antibodies. *Biotechnol. Bioeng.* **2020**, *117*, 673–686. [CrossRef]
38. Capito, F.; Skudas, R.; Kolmar, H.; Hunzinger, C. At-line mid infrared spectroscopy for monitoring downstream processing unit operations. *Process Biochem.* **2015**, *50*, 997–1005. [CrossRef]
39. Walch, N.; Scharl, T.; Felföldi, E.; Sauer, D.G.; Melcher, M.; Leisch, F.; Dürauer, A.; Jungbauer, A. Prediction of the Quantity and Purity of an Antibody Capture Process in Real Time. *Biotechnol. J.* **2019**, *14*, 1800521. [CrossRef]
40. André, S.; Cristau, L.S.; Gaillard, S.; Devos, O.; Calvosa, É.; Duponchel, L. In-line and real-time prediction of recombinant antibody titer by in situ Raman spectroscopy. *Anal. Chim. Acta* **2015**, *892*, 148–152. [CrossRef]
41. Feidl, F.; Garbellini, S.; Vogg, S.; Sokolov, M.; Souquet, J.; Broly, H.; Butté, A.; Morbidelli, M. A new flow cell and chemometric protocol for implementing in-line Raman spectroscopy in chromatography. *Biotechnol. Prog.* **2019**, *35*, e2847. [CrossRef] [PubMed]
42. Feidl, F.; Garbellini, S.; Luna, M.F.; Vogg, S.; Souquet, J.; Broly, H.; Morbidelli, M.; Butté, A. Combining Mechanistic Modeling and Raman Spectroscopy for Monitoring Antibody Chromatographic Purification. *Processes* **2019**, *7*, 683. [CrossRef]
43. Yilmaz, D.; Mehdizadeh, H.; Navarro, D.; Shehzad, A.; O'Connor, M.; McCormick, P. Application of Raman spectroscopy in monoclonal antibody producing continuous systems for downstream process intensification. *Biotechnol. Prog.* **2019**, *36*, e2947. [CrossRef]
44. Chmielowski, R.A.; Mathiasson, L.; Blom, H.; Go, D.; Ehring, H.; Khan, H.; Li, H.; Cutler, C.; Lacki, K.; Tugcu, N.; et al. Definition and dynamic control of a continuous chromatography process independent of cell culture titer and impurities. *J. Chromatogr. A* **2017**, *1526*, 58–69. [CrossRef] [PubMed]
45. Zhou, C.; Qi, W.; Lewis, E.N.; Carpenter, J.F. Concomitant Raman spectroscopy and dynamic light scattering for characterization of therapeutic proteins at high concentrations. *Anal. Biochem.* **2015**, *472*, 7–20. [CrossRef] [PubMed]
46. Gómez de la Cuesta, R.; Goodacre, R.; Ashton, L. Monitoring Antibody Aggregation in Early Drug Development Using Raman Spectroscopy and Perturbation-Correlation Moving Windows. *Anal. Chem.* **2014**, *86*, 11133–11140. [CrossRef] [PubMed]
47. Paidi, S.K.; Siddhanta, S.; Strouse, R.; McGivney, J.B.; Larkin, C.; Barman, I. Rapid Identification of Biotherapeutics with Label-Free Raman Spectroscopy. *Anal. Chem.* **2016**, *88*, 4361–4368. [CrossRef]

48. Zhang, C.; Springall, J.S.; Wang, X.; Barman, I. Rapid, quantitative determination of aggregation and particle formation for antibody drug conjugate therapeutics with label-free Raman spectroscopy. *Anal. Chim. Acta* **2019**, *1081*, 138–145. [CrossRef] [PubMed]
49. Ashton, L.; Brewster, V.L.; Correa, E.; Goodacre, R. Detection of glycosylation and iron-binding protein modifications using Raman spectroscopy. *Analyst* **2017**, *142*, 808–814. [CrossRef]
50. Brewster, V.L.; Ashton, L.; Goodacre, R. Monitoring the glycosylation status of proteins using Raman spectroscopy. *Anal. Chem.* **2011**, *83*, 6074–6081. [CrossRef]
51. Cowcher, D.P.; Deckert-Gaudig, T.; Brewster, V.L.; Ashton, L.; Deckert, V.; Goodacre, R. Detection of protein glycosylation using tip-enhanced Raman scattering. *Anal. Chem.* **2016**, *88*, 2105–2112. [CrossRef]
52. Capito, F.; Skudas, R.; Kolmar, H.; Stanislawski, B. Host cell protein quantification by fourier transform mid infrared spectroscopy (FT-MIR). *Biotechnol. Bioeng.* **2013**, *110*, 252–259. [CrossRef]
53. Virtanen, T.; Reinikainen, S.P.; Kögler, M.; Mänttäri, M.; Viitala, T.; Kallioinen, M. Real-time fouling monitoring with Raman spectroscopy. *J. Membr. Sci.* **2017**, *525*, 312–319. [CrossRef]
54. Kojima, T.; Tsutsumi, S.; Yamamoto, K.; Ikeda, Y.; Moriwaki, T. High-throughput cocrystal slurry screening by use of in situ Raman microscopy and multi-well plate. *Int. J. Pharm.* **2010**, *399*, 52–59. [CrossRef] [PubMed]
55. Medipally, D.K.; Maguire, A.; Bryant, J.; Armstrong, J.; Dunne, M.; Finn, M.; Lyng, F.M.; Meade, A.D. Development of a high throughput (HT) Raman spectroscopy method for rapid screening of liquid blood plasma from prostate cancer patients. *Analyst* **2017**, *142*, 1216–1226. [CrossRef] [PubMed]
56. Qi, J.; Shih, W.C. Performance of line-scan Raman microscopy for high-throughput chemical imaging of cell population. *Appl. Opt.* **2014**, *53*, 2881–2885. [CrossRef] [PubMed]
57. Schie, I.W.; Rüger, J.; Mondol, A.S.; Ramoji, A.; Neugebauer, U.; Krafft, C.; Popp, J. High-Throughput Screening Raman Spectroscopy Platform for Label-Free Cellomics. *Anal. Chem.* **2018**, *90*, 2023–2030. [CrossRef] [PubMed]
58. Le Losq, C. *Rampy: A Python Library for Processing Spectroscopic (IR, Raman, XAS) Data*; Zenodo: Geneva, Switzerland, 2018.
59. Wold, S.; Geladi, P.; Esbensen, K.; Öhman, J. Multi-way principal components-and PLS-analysis. *J. Chemom.* **1987**, *1*, 41–56. [CrossRef]
60. Rowland-Jones, R.C.; Jaques, C. At-line raman spectroscopy and design of experiments for robust monitoring and control of miniature bioreactor cultures. *Biotechnol. Prog.* **2019**, *35*, e2740. [CrossRef]
61. Berry, B.; Moretto, J.; Matthews, T.; Smelko, J.; Wiltberger, K. Cross-scale predictive modeling of CHO cell culture growth and metabolites using Raman spectroscopy and multivariate analysis. *Biotechnol. Prog.* **2015**, *31*, 566–577. [CrossRef]
62. Vasko, P.D.; Blackwell, J.; Koenig, J.L. Infrared and raman spectroscopy of carbohydrates: Part I: Identification of OH and CH-related vibrational modes for D-glucose, maltose, cellobiose, and dextran by deuterium-substitution methods. *Carbohydr. Res.* **1971**, *19*, 297–310. [CrossRef]
63. Mathlouthi, M.; Vinh Luu, D. Laser-raman spectra of d-glucose and sucrose in aqueous solution. *Carbohydr. Res.* **1980**, *81*, 203–212. [CrossRef]
64. Söderholm, S.; Roos, Y.H.; Meinander, N.; Hotokka, M. Raman spectra of fructose and glucose in the amorphous and crystalline states. *J. Raman Spectrosc.* **1999**, *30*, 1009–1018. [CrossRef]
65. Singh, G.P.; Goh, S.; Canzoneri, M.; Ram, R.J. Raman spectroscopy of complex defined media: Biopharmaceutical applications. *J. Raman Spectrosc.* **2015**, *46*, 545–550. [CrossRef]
66. Barrett, T.W. Laser Raman spectra of mono-, oligo- and polysaccharides in solution. *Spectrochim. Acta Part A Mol. Spectrosc.* **1981**, *37*, 233–239. [CrossRef]
67. De Gelder, J.; De Gussem, K.; Vandenabeele, P.; Moens, L. Reference database of Raman spectra of biological molecules. *J. Raman Spectrosc.* **2007**, *38*, 1133–1147. [CrossRef]
68. Kačuráková, M.; Mathlouthi, M. FTIR and laser-Raman spectra of oligosaccharides in water: Characterization of the glycosidic bond. *Carbohydr. Res.* **1996**, *284*, 145–157. [CrossRef]
69. Rhiel, M.H.; Amrhein, M.I.; Marison, I.W.; Stockar, U. The Influence of Correlated Calibration Samples on the Prediction Performance of Multivariate Models Based on Mid-Infrared Spectra of Animal Cell Cultures. *Anal. Chem.* **2002**, *74*, 5227–5236. [CrossRef]
70. Cassanas, G.; Morssli, M.; Fabregue, E.; Bardet, L. Vibrational spectra of lactic acid and lactates. *J. Raman Spectrosc.* **1991**, *22*, 409–413. [CrossRef]

71. Pecul, M.; Rizzo, A.; Leszczynski, J. Vibrational Raman and Raman Optical Activity Spectra of d-Lactic Acid, d-Lactate, and d-Glyceraldehyde: Ab Initio Calculations. *J. Phys. Chem. A* **2002**, *106*, 11008–11016. [CrossRef]
72. Kengne-Momo, R.P.; Daniel, P.; Lagarde, F.; Jeyachandran, Y.L.; Pilard, J.F.; Durand-Thouand, M.J.; Thouand, G. Protein interactions investigated by the Raman spectroscopy for biosensor applications. *Int. J. Spectrosc.* **2012**, *2012*, 462901. [CrossRef]
73. Painter, P.C.; Koenig, J.L. Raman spectroscopic study of the structure of antibodies. *Biopolymers* **1975**, *14*, 457–468. [CrossRef]
74. Carey, P.R. CHAPTER 4—Protein Conformation from Raman and Resonance Raman Spectra. In *Biochemical Applications of Raman and Resonance Raman Spectroscopes*; Carey, P.R., Ed.; Academic Press: Cambridge, MA, USA, 1982; pp. 71–98.

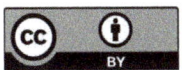

© 2020 by the authors. Licensee MDPI, Basel, Switzerland. This article is an open access article distributed under the terms and conditions of the Creative Commons Attribution (CC BY) license (http://creativecommons.org/licenses/by/4.0/).

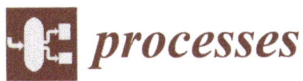

Article

Real-Time Nanoplasmonic Sensor for IgG Monitoring in Bioproduction

Thuy Tran [1], Olof Eskilson [1], Florian Mayer [2], Robert Gustavsson [2], Robert Selegård [1], Ingemar Lundström [3], Carl-Fredrik Mandenius [2], Erik Martinsson [4] and Daniel Aili [1,*]

1. Laboratory of Molecular Materials, Division of Biophysics and Bioengineering, Department of Physics, Chemistry and Biology, Linköping University, 581 83 Linköping, Sweden; thuy.tran@liu.se (T.T.); olof.eskilsson@liu.se (O.E.); robert.selegard@liu.se (R.S.)
2. Laboratory of Biotechnology, Division of Biophysics and Bioengineering, Department of Physics, Chemistry and Biology, Linköping University, 581 83 Linköping, Sweden; florian.mayer1994@gmx.at (F.M.); robert.gustavsson@liu.se (R.G.); carl-fredrik.mandenius@liu.se (C.-F.M.)
3. Sensor and Actuator Systems, Department of Physics, Chemistry and Biology, Linköping University, 581 83 Linköping, Sweden; ingemar.lundstrom@liu.se
4. ArgusEye AB, Spannmålsgatan 55, 583 36 Linköping, Sweden; erik.martinsson@arguseye.se
* Correspondence: daniel.aili@liu.se

Received: 21 September 2020; Accepted: 14 October 2020; Published: 16 October 2020

Abstract: Real-time monitoring of product titers during process development and production of biotherapeutics facilitate implementation of quality-by-design principles and enable rapid bioprocess decision and optimization of the production process. Conventional analytical methods are generally performed offline/at-line and, therefore, are not capable of generating real-time data. In this study, a novel fiber optical nanoplasmonic sensor technology was explored for rapid IgG titer measurements. The sensor combines localized surface plasmon resonance transduction and robust single use Protein A-modified sensor chips, housed in a flexible flow cell, for specific IgG detection. The sensor requires small sample volumes (1–150 µL) and shows a reproducibility and sensitivity comparable to Protein G high performance liquid chromatography-ultraviolet (HPLC-UV). The dynamic range of the sensor system can be tuned by varying the sample volume, which enables quantification of IgG samples ranging from 0.0015 to 10 mg/mL, without need for sample dilution. The sensor shows limited interference from the sample matrix and negligible unspecific protein binding. IgG titers can be rapidly determined in samples from filtered unpurified Chinese hamster ovary (CHO) cell cultures and show good correlation with enzyme-linked immunosorbent assay (ELISA).

Keywords: PAT; IgG titer; real-time; on-line; bioprocess; nanoplasmonic

---

1. Introduction

Efficient and cost-effective production of biologics requires the ability to accurately monitor and control the production process. Guidelines concerning process analytical technologies (PATs) released by the U.S. Food and Drug Administration (FDA) in 2004 [1] initiated a large interest in development and implementation of technologies for near real-time or real-time monitoring of key performance indicators (KPIs) and critical quality attributes (CQAs) in bioproduction [2–4].

Therapeutic antibodies are currently the largest group of biopharmaceuticals. Until 2019, a total of 79 therapeutic immunoglobulin G (IgG) monoclonal antibodies (mAbs) had been approved by the U.S. FDA [5,6]. Techniques for process development and production of mAbs using mammalian cell cultures have been evolving rapidly, resulting in product titers ranging from about 1 to 10 mg/mL using CHO cell cultures [7–10]. Possibilities to monitor IgG titers are central for optimizing process conditions and to achieve high yields as well as consistent and high product quality. The IgG titer is thus naturally an important KPI in production of mAbs. There are several techniques that can be used for measuring IgG titers, such as enzyme-linked immunosorbent assay (ELISA) [11], protein A/G high performance liquid chromatography-ultraviolet (Protein A/G-HPLC-UV) [12,13], surface plasmon resonance (SPR) [14,15], biolayer interferometry (BLI) [16] and capillary electrophoresis-mass spectrometry (CE-MS) [17]. Among these, protein A/G-HPLC-UV has been the most widely used method for bioprocess monitoring and validation due to its high selectivity, robustness and reliable results. However, these methods typically require multiple sample preparation steps and are difficult to automize and implement as on-line/in-line techniques and are, therefore, generally performed at-line or off-line. Possibilities to acquire specific near real-time or real-time data of IgG titers are thus limited. With the increasing demand for applying PAT tools in bioprocessing, efforts have been made to reduce the turn-around time of available analytical methods. Pedersen et al. introduced a method using flow-induced dispersion analysis that could quantify IgG in cell culture broth in less than 15 min [18]. Swartz et al. developed a quick and cost-effective antibody-nanocage turbidity assay for rapid measurements of IgG in cell culture samples [19]. These methodologies were, however, not possible to integrate for on-line measurements. An on-line/at-line system using a portable ultraperformance liquid chromatography (UPLC) system interfaced with an UPLC–process sample manager was recently developed by Letha et al., indicating the potential for more rapid IgG titer measurements [20]. The technique, however, requires complex equipment and sample handling, including purification, which complicates implementation in bioproduction. Despite large efforts to improve the speed of IgG quantification methods, there is still a lack of robust cost-effective sensor systems that allow for specific on-line real-time titer measurements.

Localized surface plasmon resonance (LSPR)-based sensors, or nanoplasmonic sensors, have emerged as versatile techniques for label-free biomolecular interaction analysis [21–23]. LSPR is an optical phenomenon caused by coherent electron oscillations in metal nanostructures. The resonance conditions are sensitive to changes in refractive index in the immediate vicinity of the nanostructures, which enable detection of analyte binding to immobilized ligands. In comparison to benchtop surface plasmon resonance (SPR) sensor systems, LSPR sensors require significantly less complex optical setups and are less sensitive to temperature fluctuations and changes in the sample background. However, SPR can enable label-free at-line and off-line monitoring of IgG titers in samples from upstream process steps but, due to the narrow and low dynamic range, with reported values spanning from 13–30 µg/mL [24], 0.019–9.6 µg/mL [15] to 2–200 µg/mL [14], extensive sample dilution is required.

Here, we explore a novel LSPR-based sensor technology that combines nanoplasmonic sensing with fiber optics that is possible to integrate for specific on-line/in-line biodetection in real-time. The sensor technology, schematically described in Figure 1, was developed in close collaboration with ArgusEye AB (Linköping, Sweden) with the purpose of enabling more efficient bioprocess monitoring. To our knowledge this is the first LSPR-based sensor system designed for on-line/in-line bioprocess monitoring. The analytical performance of the sensor system for detection of IgG in complex samples was evaluated using samples from both upstream and downstream process steps, and data was in good agreement with results from ELISA and protein G-HPLC-UV. The sensor has a short response time (seconds to minutes) and a large and tunable dynamic range (from 0.0015 mg/mL to about 30 mg/mL) and was capable of rapid IgG quantification in cell-free samples directly without any need for sample pretreatment. Successful integration of this novel sensor technology in bioproduction and process development could improve process understanding, facilitate implementation of quality by design (QbD) and development of strategies for continuous processing.

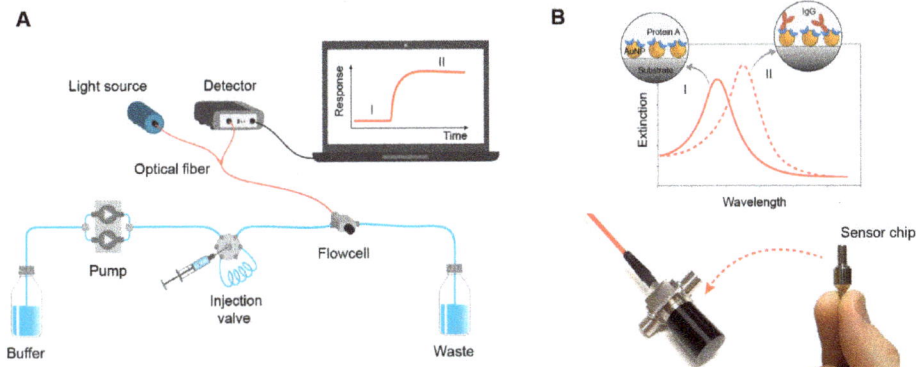

Figure 1. (**A**) Schematic illustration of the sensor system setup. Samples with IgG were injected into the flow cell containing the sensor chip. (**B**) Nanoplasmonic sensor chips were functionalized with Protein A for specific recognition of IgG. Binding of IgG to the sensor chip results in a concentration-dependent redshift of the LSPR peak maximum. The sensor signal is transmitted to the detector using fiber optics and was monitored in real-time using a dedicated software.

2. Materials and Methods

2.1. Chemicals and Reagents

N-Ethyl-N'-(3-dimethylaminopropyl)carbodiimide (EDC), N-Hydroxysuccinimide (NHS), Bovine serum albumin (BSA), ethanolamine, 4-Morpholineethanesulfonic acid (MES), purified IgG from human serum (5.5 g/L) were obtained from Sigma-Aldrich (St. Louis, MO, USA). Protein A was supplied by Medicago AB (Upsala, Sweden). Hyclone ActiPro Medium, Hyclone Cell boost 7a, Hyclone Cell boost 7b were purchased from GE Healthcare Life Sciences (Logan, UT, USA). Sheep antihuman IgG gamma chain and sheep antihuman IgG gamma chain peroxidase conjugate were purchased from by The Binding Site Group Ltd (Birmingham, UK). TMB (Tetramethylbenzidine) substrate kit, Novex sharp prestained protein standard, Bolt LDS sample buffer, Bolt 4–12% Bis-Tris Plus gels, MOPS (4-Morpholinepropanesulfonic acid) SDS running buffer, SimplyBlue SafeStain solution were purchased from Thermo Fisher Scientific (Rockford, IL, USA). GlutaMAX™ (100×) was from Life Technologies/Gibco (Carlsbad, CA, USA).

2.2. Ligand Immobilization

Ligand immobilization to carboxyl sensor chips (ArgusEye AB, Linköping, Sweden) was carried out using carbodiimide (EDC/NHS) coupling chemistry. A (v/v 1:1) mixture of 20 µL of 0.4 M EDC and 0.1 M NHS was added to the sensor surfaces, and carboxyl groups were activated for 45 min. After rinsing with Milli-Q water (18.2 MΩ cm^{-1}), 20 µL of 0.5 mg/mL ligand solution was added and the coupling reaction was carried out for 2 h. Unreacted carboxyl groups were deactivated by using of 20 µL of 1 M ethanolamine (pH 8.5) for 30 min. The sensor substrates were rinsed and stored in PBS buffer before being inserted into the LSPR system.

2.3. LSPR Measurements

The fiber optical sensor system was provided by ArgusEye AB and includes a flow cell and an optical detection unit comprising a halogen light source and a spectrophotometer. Sensor chips functionalized with Protein A (ProtA) or BSA were inserted into the flow cell and equilibrated with PBS buffer at a flow rate of 1 mL/min using an HPLC pump for about 15 min to ensure stable baseline. Samples were manually injected into the flow cell and the sensor signal was continuously recorded using software developed by ArgusEye. Purified monomeric IgG and filtrated bioreactor samples (provided by BioInvent International AB, Lund, Sweden) were used to validate the analytical performance of the sensor system. The system was run in a normal laboratory setting at room temperature without any additional temperature control.

2.4. CHO Cell Cultivation

A recombinant CHO cell line (CHOK-1 derivate cell line) producing human IgG was provided from Cobra Biologics Ltd. (Newcastle, UK). The CHO cell line was cultured in spinner flasks in fed-batch mode at 37 °C in a humidified atmosphere containing 7.5% CO_2. HyClone Actipro™ medium supplemented with 3% GlutaMAX™ (100×) was used as culture media. At day three of culture, a daily feed of 2% HyClone Cell Boost™ 7a and 0.2% HyClone Cell Boost™ 7b of the culture volume was applied. Samples for analysis were withdrawn from the culture daily, centrifuged (200× g, 5 min) and the supernatant was 0.2 µm filtered before storage at −20 °C.

2.5. ELISA IgG Quantification

ELISA assays were performed using a general colorimetric sandwich ELISA procedure. Briefly, Sheep antihuman IgG gamma chain was coated on a Maxisorp Nunc-Immuno well plate (Thermo Fisher Scientific) and incubated overnight at 4 °C. After rinsing, standards (Purified IgG from human serum) and samples were added and incubated for 2 h at 37 °C. Samples were discarded followed by adding sheep antihuman IgG gamma chain peroxidase conjugate and incubated for 1 h at 37 °C. Color development using TMB solution was done at room temperature and the reaction was stopped using H_2SO_4. Absorbances at 450 nm and 620 nm were measured for quantification.

2.6. SDS-PAGE IgG Quantification

Novex sharp prestained protein standards were used as molecular weight standards. Samples and standards (Purified IgG from human serum) were mixed with Bolt LDS sample buffer and purified water and incubated for 10 min at 70 °C. The samples were loaded on Bolt 4–12% Bis-Tris Plus gels, and electrophoresis was performed at 200 V for between 35 to 45 min using an XCell SureLock electrophoresis cell (Thermo Fisher Scientific, Carlsbad, CA, USA) and a E443 power supply (Consort). Bolt MOPS SDS running buffer was used as running buffer. Gels were stained by using SimplyBlue SafeStain solution with 1 h incubation and destained using purified water for 1 h. The gels were scanned for further evaluation and quantification.

3. Results and Discussion

3.1. LSPR Detection Setup

The LSPR measurements were conducted using a novel fiber optical sensor system comprised of a flow cell designed for real-time on-line and in-line bioproduction monitoring connected to a halogen light source and a detector using fiber optics (Figure 1). The flow cell was produced in medical grade stainless steel to tolerate both cleaning in place and high pressures. Single use sensor chips, modified with gold nanostructures and functionalized with Protein A, were docked into the flow cell to enable specific IgG detection. Analyte binding results in a change in refractive index detected as a shift in the LSPR resonance conditions. The sensor response (in picometer, pm) was recorded in real time and the sensorgrams indicated both analyte concentration and binding kinetics. To simulate on-line conditions, the flow cell was connected to a manual injection valve. An HPLC pump was used to control the flow, and samples were injected into the flow cell using an injection valve with replaceable sample loops with different volumes. In a real on-line detection setup, this would be replaced by an automated system where sample fractions are collected using software-controlled valves.

3.2. Protein A Immobilization

The sensor chips were fabricated in medical grade stainless steel modified with nanoplasmonic gold nanostructures and further functionalized with a robust surface chemistry that enables covalent immobilization of ligands using carbodiimide chemistry. The pH of the coupling buffer influences both the net charge of ProtA (pI (isoeletric point) = 5.1) and the net-charge of the sensor surface, which can affect the electrostatic attraction between the sensor surface and the protein during the coupling reaction. ProtA with a concentration of 0.5 mg/mL prepared in three different buffers, acetate pH 4.0, MES pH 6.0, and phosphate buffer pH 7.0 was used to compare the influence of pH on coupling efficiency (Appendix A, Figure A1). The acidic buffers were found to give only marginally higher IgG binding responses compared to neutral pH, which indicated that the effect of pH in this case was not significant. ProtA immobilization was, therefore, conducted using 10 mM MES pH 6.0 in all further experiments.

3.3. Sensor Evaluation

3.3.1. Unspecific Binding

The binding of IgG to the ProtA sensor chips was investigated using a simulated on-line setup where samples were manually injected into the sensor flow system using an HPLC injection port. Injection of IgG (1 mg/mL) resulted in an LSPR response of about 2000 pm (Figure 2A,B). In contrast, when using bovine serum albumin (BSA) as a ligand instead of ProtA, no significant binding could be detected (Figure 2A,B). The contribution from unspecific binding of IgG to the sensor signal was consequently below the detection limit of the sensor. When injecting undiluted cell culture media (1 mL) to a ProtA chip, a negative response was obtained, followed by a very small increase in the baseline, corresponding to only about 2% of the specific IgG binding. The negative shift is a consequence of the yellow color of the cell culture medium that interferes with the baseline. After the injection has passed through the flow cell, the baseline stabilizes and returns to normal. Consequently, the readout of protein binding to sensor surface must, in this case, be assessed after the injection. Here, the responses during the dissociation phase (t > 150 s, 40.6 pm) better reflect the binding and indicate a negligible unspecific interaction between components in the cell culture medium and the ProtA sensor chip (Figure 2B). The negative dip can also, if needed, be subtracted by including a reference cell to the system. In these experiments, the sample volume was 1 mL and was injected into the system at a flow rate of 1 mL/min. With smaller sample volumes, the influence of sample color can be eliminated and effects of unspecific binding further reduced (vide infra).

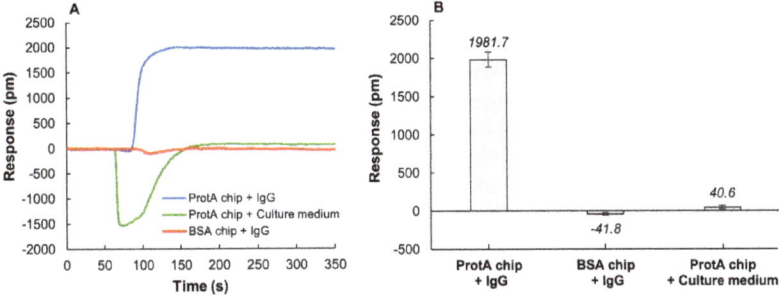

Figure 2. Unspecific binding evaluation using bovine serum albumin (BSA) chips and cell culture medium (HyClone ActiPro™ + GlutaMax) as negative controls. (**A**) Representative sensorgrams showing the binding of IgG (1 mg/mL) to a ProtA chip and a BSA chip, and the binding of cell culture medium to a ProtA chip. (**B**) Comparison of specific and unspecific binding responses. Relative binding responses at t = 250 s were averaged (n = 3 sensor chips), and error bars show standard deviations. Injection volume was 1 mL.

3.3.2. Regeneration Scouting

As in most other affinity-based biosensors, the ProtA sensor chips can be regenerated to allow for multiple consecutive measurements. To evaluate the efficiency of the regeneration process, different concentrations of IgG were injected followed by a short (1 min) 10 mM glycine buffer pH 2.5 pulse (Figure 3A). The regeneration buffer efficiently disrupted the interaction between IgG and ProtA and the signal returned to baseline after a single regeneration pulse for the two lower (0.0625 and 0.156 mg/mL) IgG concentrations. After a second regeneration pulse, the chip exposed to 1 mg/mL IgG also returned close to baseline (Figure 3A,B). ProtA is fairly stable under these conditions but to verify the effect of the regeneration buffer on the IgG binding, eight cycles of IgG injections, each followed by two regeneration pulses, were conducted (Figure 3C). Absolute and relative binding responses at the last injection were reduced by only 1.5 and 4.8%, respectively, as compared to the first injection (Figure 3D). The ProtA chips are, consequently, both robust enough to allow for multiple consecutive measurements while efficiently preventing unspecific protein binding, which are important properties for PAT applications.

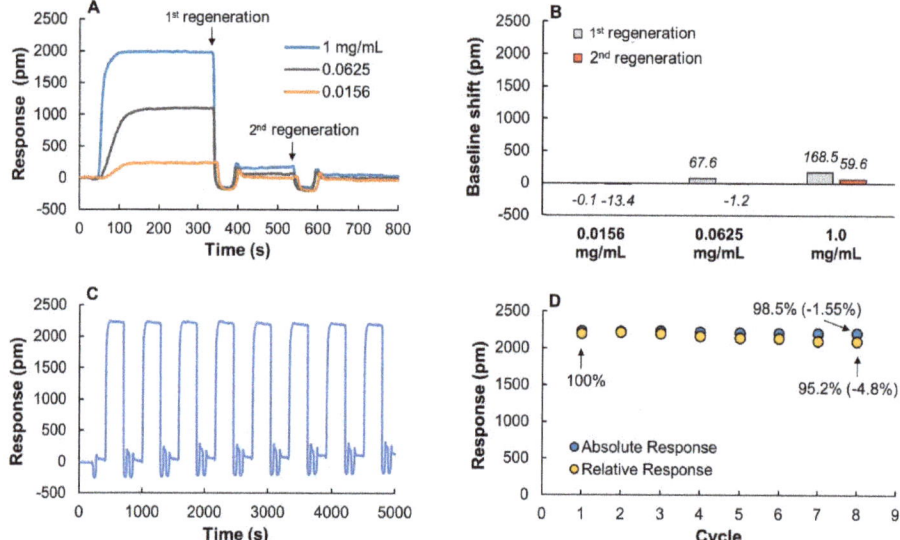

Figure 3. (**A**) Binding and regeneration profiles of IgG to a ProtA chip using three IgG concentrations: 0.0156, 0.0625 and 1 mg/mL. (**B**) Baseline shift after first and second regeneration pulse. (**C**) Sensorgrams obtained after eight cycles of IgG injections (1 mg/mL) each followed by two regeneration pulses using 10 mM glycine buffer pH 2.5. (**D**) Change in absolute and relative binding responses after each binding and regeneration cycle. The relative binding response is the difference between the absolute responses and the baseline before each IgG injection. The sample volume was 1 mL in all experiments.

3.3.3. IgG Binding Reproducibility

To test the reproducibility and robustness of the sensor system, binding responses from three different sensor chips were compared using IgG samples with different concentrations: 0.0156, 0.0625 and 2 mg/mL (Figure 4). The colored area in the sensorgrams indicate the 95% confidence intervals for three independent sensor chips and two injection replicates per chip. Binding responses at t = 250 s were used to evaluate the variation between sensor chips and within sensor chips. Coefficient of variation (CV) of the binding responses across sensor chips varied from 9.5 to 12.7%, while with the same chip, the variations were only about 3 to 4% (Table 1). These results show that the data generated using the sensor system were highly reproducible, also when using different sensor chips.

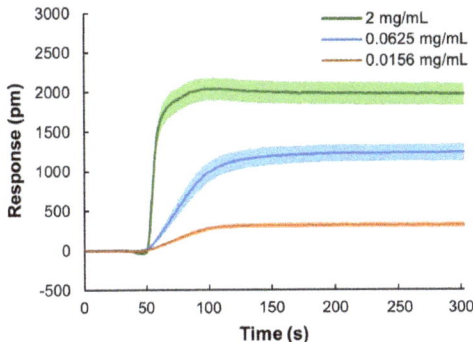

Figure 4. Evaluation of reproducibility of sensor chips. Mean responses from six runs using n = 3 different chips and two injection replicates per chip using three different IgG concentrations, 0.0156, 0.0625 and 2 mg/mL. The data show 95% confidence intervals. Injection volume was 1 mL.

Table 1. Coefficient of variation (CV) of binding responses at t = 250 s of three IgG concentrations: 0.015, 0.0625 and 2 mg/mL. Between-chip CV was calculated based on the mean responses obtained from three different chips. Within-chip CV was the mean of CV calculated based on binding responses obtained from the same chip.

Concentration (mg/mL)	0.0156	0.0625	2
Between-Chip CV (%)	12.7	11.4	9.5
Within-Chip CV (%)	2.6	3.3	4.3

3.3.4. Dynamic Range

The ProtA sensor chips have a certain number of accessible IgG binding sites that depend on the surface concentration of immobilized ProtA and their relative orientation on the sensor surface and, therefore, show an upper limit in binding capacity. When fully saturated, the sensor response was about 2000 pm. The IgG concentration required to saturate the surface was found to depend on injection volume (Appendix A, Figure A2), which enables flexible tuning of the dynamic range. The dynamic range of the sensor system was investigated using three different injection volumes, 1 mL, 20 µL and 1 µL. The sensor surface was saturated at lower concentrations when increasing the injection volumes (Figure 5). By varying the injection volume in the range of 1 µL to 1 mL, the total dynamic range could be expanded to more than three orders of magnitude, from 0.0015 to about 30 mg/mL. The linear range for quantification was estimated to be 0.0015–0.06, 0.125–1.5, and 0.5–10 mg/mL at 1 mL, 20 µL and 1 µL injection volumes, respectively. Compared to ELISA [25,26], which is normally performed at the µg/mL level, and to a recently developed protein A-HPLC-UV method [27] with an improved linear range of 0.01–5.2 mg/mL, the sensor system used here showed a substantially higher upper limit for quantification. The linear range reported in present work covers the range of normal cell culture titers (5–10 mg/mL) that can be routinely achieved in industrial cell culture processes nowadays [7,8]. Therefore, bioreactor samples can be analyzed without the need of dilution, which simplifies sample handling and facilitates on-line/in-line detection.

3.3.5. IgG Quantification in Bioreactor Samples

Filtrated crude bioreactor samples, provided from an industrial bioproduction process with a known concentration of 2.3 mg/mL determined by Protein G-HPLC-UV, were used to validate the method for quantification. Nine IgG standards diluted from a monomeric sample of the same IgG were used to calibrate the system, and two injections of sample were used for concentration determination. A full recording of both standards and samples are shown in Figure 6A. Extracted sensorgrams of IgG concentrations, 0.5, 1, 2, 3, 5, and 10 mg/mL defining the linear range are shown in Figure 6B. Interestingly, although the bioreactor samples had a distinct yellow color, the negative dip seen during the association phase when using 1 mL injection volumes (Figure 2A) was not observed here when using a smaller sample volume of 1 µL. The linearity of the standard curve was high with $R^2 = 0.9962$, and the determined concentration of 2.5 mg/mL was in very good agreement with the expected value (Figure 6C).

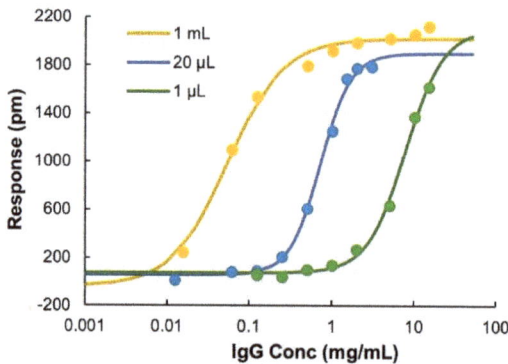

Figure 5. Binding responses at t = 250 s versus IgG concentrations fitted to sigmoidal curves when using various sample injection volumes, 1 µL, 20 µL, and 1 mL.

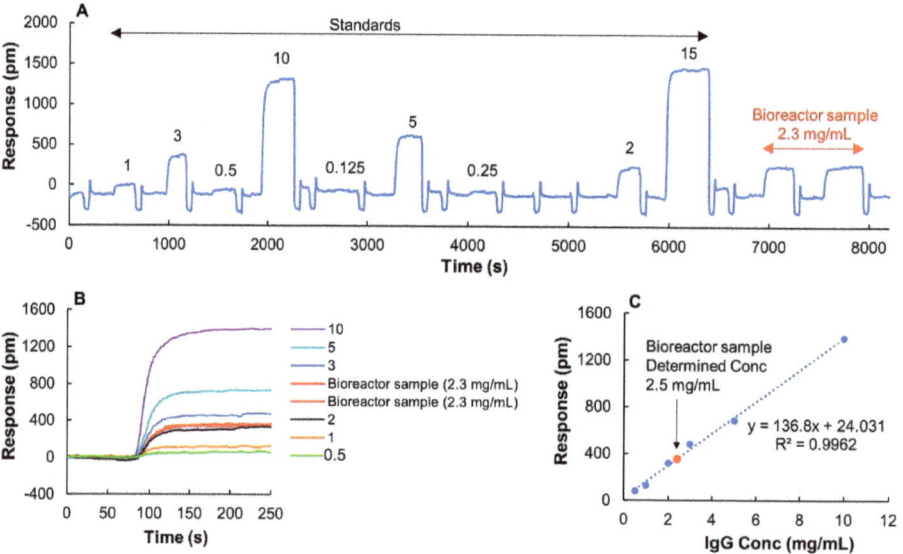

Figure 6. Quantification of IgG in filtrated upstream samples from a bioreactor cell culture. The sample has an IgG concentration of 2.3 mg/mL determined by traditional Protein G-HPLC-UV. (**A**) A full run of nine IgG standards with various concentrations starting from 0.125 to 15 mg/mL and two injections of the bioreactor sample. 1 µL of samples was used for measurements. Concentrations are displayed on top of each individual sensorgram. The sensor chip was regenerated using 10 mM glycine buffer pH 2.5 after each sample injection. (**B**) Extracted and normalized sensorgrams of the sample and six IgG standards (0.5, 1, 2, 3, 5, 10 mg/mL) used for making the calibration curve. (**C**) Calibration curve and determined concentration of sample based on two replicates.

3.4. Measurement of IgG Titers during Cell Culture

The possibility to rapidly and accurately determine IgG titers over a wide concentration range in an upstream process step was further assessed using a CHO fed-batch culture. Samples collected daily for 15 days from a CHO cell culture were measured using the same sensor chip and IgG titers were determined. A full run, including standards and samples, is shown in Figure 7A. Negative dips in the sensorgrams of samples (D0–D14) were caused by the color of the media but did not interfere with the analysis of the data. Based on the linear range (Figure 7B) and expected concentrations of IgG, a sample volume of 150 µL was used for all the measurements. The binding responses leveled off at day 11 (Figure 7C), indicating that a maximum titer was achieved. Since the binding responses of samples at day 11, 12, 13 and 14 were lower than the maximum binding capacity (2036 ± 120 pm), and were within the linear range of the sensor chip, the sensor surface was never saturated.

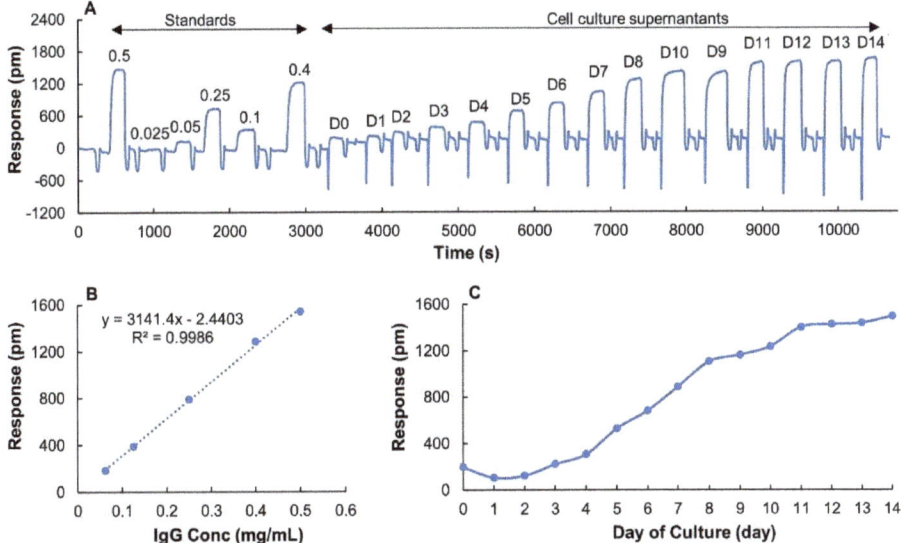

Figure 7. LSPR measurement of filtrated cell culture samples collected daily over two weeks of cultivation. (**A**) A full run of six IgG standards (diluted from downstream monomeric IgG sample 15 mg/mL) with different concentrations marked on top of each sensorgram and 15 cell culture samples collected from day 0 to day 14 (D0–D14). Injection volume was 150 µL. (**B**) Calibration curve. (**C**) Binding responses of samples over cultivation time.

In Figure 8A, the LSPR data are compared to results from ELISA and SDS-PAGE. All methods show a similar trend, that the highest IgG titers were reached at around day 10–11. There was no significant difference between ELISA and LSPR titers for 13 of the 15 measured samples. Titers estimated using ELISA in samples from day 10 and 11 were higher compared to LSPR. For ELISA, there was a drop in IgG titers after day 11. However, such change was not seen in either LSPR or SDS-PAGE. Interestingly, ELISA gave higher IgG titers than LSPR for day 10 and 11 but the same titers as LSPR after that. The ELISA titers were, therefore, likely overestimated for these two samples. Despite this difference, a high degree of correlation ($R^2 = 0.9629$) between these two methods was obtained using linear regression analysis (Figure 8B). The growth curve from LSPR also showed good correlation with SDS-PAGE (sodium dodecyl sulfate-polyacrylamide gel electrophoresis) and a similar correlation coefficient was attained as when comparing LSPR and ELISA. Both ELISA and LSPR use ligand specificity for IgG detection. The small variation in IgG titers between the two methods could be a result of different IgG ligands used for the calibrations. Binding of Human IgG to Anti-human IgG gamma chain and monomeric recombinant IgG to Protein A were used for ELISA and LSPR calibration, respectively. Ideally, for both methods, the sample and the standard should contain the same type of IgG.

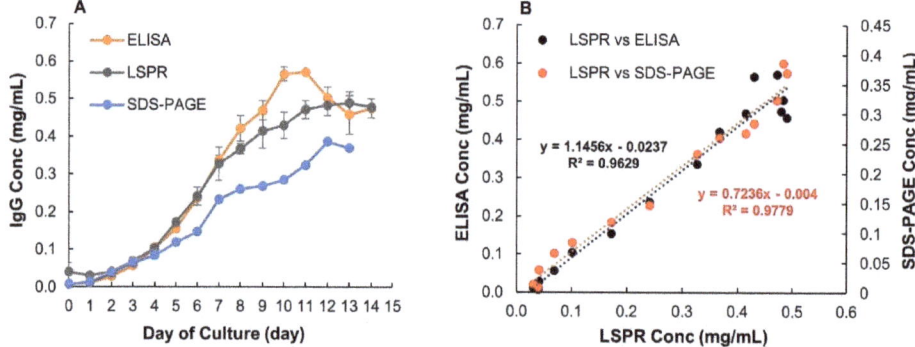

Figure 8. (**A**) Comparison of IgG titers over cultivation time obtained by ELISA, SDS-PAGE and the developed LSPR sensor. Error bars represent standard deviations (n = 3 and 2 for ELISA and LSPR, respectively. (**B**) Scatter plot and linear regression analysis for comparison of LSPR versus ELISA and LSPR versus SDS-PAGE.

4. Conclusions

In the present work, a reproducible and reliable nanoplasmonic sensor system for rapid monitoring of IgG titers was evaluated. IgG quantification results from crude cell culture supernatants were highly comparable to conventional protein G-HPLC-UV and ELISA methods. The sample measurement was completed within two minutes by injecting filtrated crude samples directly into the sensor system. The linear dynamic detection range could also be tuned by varying the injection volumes, and samples with concentrations from 0.0015 up to 10 mg/mL could be quantified. The large dynamic range enabled monitoring of titers commonly seen in both upstream and downstream process steps without any sample dilution. While all the measurements in this work were performed under simulated on-line conditions, the flexible sensor design can enable real-time operation on-line when combined with an auto-sampler that diverts or collects and directs cell-free samples from bioreactors into the flow cell. We thus envision that this novel sensor system can be utilized as a versatile technology for on-line real-time IgG monitoring in both process development and bioproduction.

Author Contributions: Conceptualization, D.A., I.L., C.-F.M. and E.M.; methodology, T.T., O.E., E.M., F.M.; software, E.M.; formal analysis, T.T., E.M., D.A.; investigation, T.T., O.E.; writing—original draft preparation, T.T.; writing—review and editing, D.A., T.T., I.L., C.-F.M., E.M., O.E., R.G., R.S., F.M.; supervision, D.A.; funding acquisition, D.A. All authors have read and agreed to the published version of the manuscript.

Funding: This research was funded by the European Union's Horizon 2020 research and innovation program under the Marie Skłodowska-Curie grant agreement No. 841373 and the Swedish Innovation Agency (VINNOVA), grant numbers 2016-04120 and 2019-00130.

Acknowledgments: Funding from the European Union's Horizon 2020 research and innovation program under the Marie Skłodowska-Curie grant agreement No. 841373 and the Swedish Innovation Agency (VINNOVA), grant numbers 2016-04120 and 2019-00130, are gratefully acknowledged.

Conflicts of Interest: D.A., E.M., I.L. and C.-F.M. are cofounders of ArgusEye AB.

Appendix A

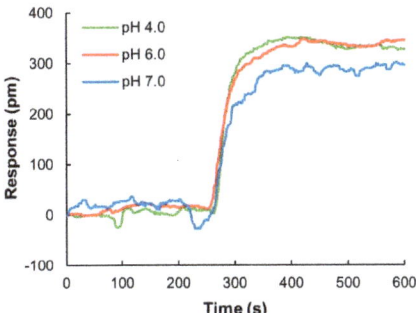

Figure A1. pH scouting for surface functionalization using glass sensor chips that have the same surface chemistry as stainless-steel chips. Protein A was immobilized to the sensor surface using 10 mM sodium acetate pH 4.0, 10 mM MES pH 6.0 and 10 mM phosphate buffer pH 7.0.

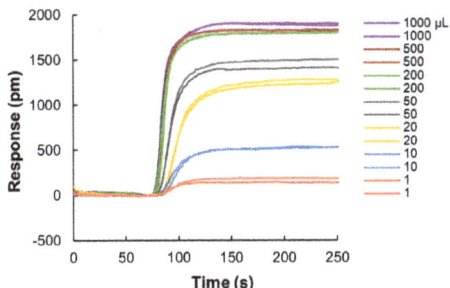

Figure A2. Binding responses of IgG sample (1 mg/mL) at different injection volumes ranging from 1 µL to 1 mL. For injection volumes > 200 µL, the responses reached maximum binding capacity of the sensor chip. Sensorgrams of two replicates of each injection volumes are depicted with the same color.

References

1. PAT—A Framework for Innovative Pharmaceutical Development, Manufacturing, and Quality Assurance. 2004. Available online: https://www.fda.gov/media/71012/download (accessed on 29 August 2020).
2. Rathore, A.S.; Bhambure, R.; Ghare, V. Process analytical technology (PAT) for biopharmaceutical products. *Anal. Bioanal. Chem.* **2010**, *398*, 137–154. [CrossRef]
3. Glassey, J.; Gernaey, K.V.; Clemens, C.; Schulz, T.W.; Oliveira, R.; Striedner, G.; Mandenius, C.F. Process analytical technology (PAT) for biopharmaceuticals. *Biotechnol. J.* **2011**, *6*, 369–377. [CrossRef]
4. Guerra, A.; Von Stosch, M.; Glassey, J. Toward biotherapeutic product real-time quality monitoring. *Crit. Rev. Biotechnol.* **2019**, *39*, 289–305. [CrossRef]
5. Kesik-Brodacka, M. Progress in biopharmaceutical development. *Biotechnol. Appl. Biochem.* **2018**, *65*, 306–322. [CrossRef]
6. Tsumoto, K.; Isozaki, Y.; Yagami, H.; Tomita, M. Future perspectives of therapeutic monoclonal antibodies. *Immunotherapy* **2019**, *11*, 119–127. [CrossRef] [PubMed]
7. Shukla, A.A.; Wolfe, L.S.; Mostafa, S.S.; Norman, C. Evolving trends in mAb production processes. *Bioeng. Transl. Med.* **2017**, *2*, 58–69. [CrossRef] [PubMed]
8. Kunert, R.; Reinhart, D. Advances in recombinant antibody manufacturing. *Appl. Microbiol. Biotechnol.* **2016**, *100*, 3451–3461. [CrossRef] [PubMed]
9. Huang, Y.-M.; Hu, W.; Rustandi, E.; Chang, K.; Yusuf-Makagiansar, H.; Ryll, T. Maximizing productivity of CHO cell-based fed-batch culture using chemically defined media conditions and typical manufacturing equipment. *Biotechnol. Prog.* **2010**, *26*, 1400–1410. [CrossRef] [PubMed]

10. Reinhart, D.; Damjanovic, L.; Kaisermayer, C.; Kunert, R. Benchmarking of commercially available CHO cell culture media for antibody production. *Appl. Microbiol. Biotechnol.* **2015**, *99*, 4645–4657. [CrossRef]
11. Mushens, R.E.; Guest, A.R.; Scott, M.L. Quantitation of monoclonal antibodies by ELISA: The use of purified mouse IgG and mouse IgM monoclonal antibodies as standards in a quantitative ELISA measuring monoclonal antibodies produced by cell culture. *J. Immunol. Methods* **1993**, *162*, 77–83. [CrossRef]
12. Horak, J.; Ronacher, A.; Lindner, W. Quantification of immunoglobulin G and characterization of process related impurities using coupled Protein A and size exclusion high performance liquid chromatography. *J. Chromatogr. A* **2010**, *1217*, 5092–5102. [CrossRef] [PubMed]
13. Fernández, L.P.; Calvo, L.; Viña, L. Development and Validation of an Affinity Chromatography-Protein G Method for IgG Quantification. *Int. Sch. Res. Not.* **2014**, *2014*, 48710. [CrossRef]
14. Frostell, Å.; Mattsson, A.; Eriksson, Å.; Wallby, E.; Kärnhall, J.; Illarionova, N.B.; Nilsson, C.E. Nine surface plasmon resonance assays for specific protein quantitation during cell culture and process development. *Anal. Biochem.* **2015**, *477*, 1–9. [CrossRef]
15. Zschätzsch, M.; Ritter, P.; Henseleit, A.; Wiehler, K.; Malik, S.; Bley, T.; Walther, T.; Boschke, E. Monitoring bioactive and total antibody concentrations for continuous process control by surface plasmon resonance spectroscopy. *Eng. Life Sci.* **2019**, *19*, 681–690. [CrossRef]
16. Yu, Y.; Mitchell, S.; Lynaugh, H.; Brown, M.; Nobrega, R.P.; Zhi, X.; Sun, T.; Caffry, I.; Cao, Y.; Yang, R.; et al. Understanding ForteBio's Sensors for High-Throughput Kinetic and Epitope Screening for Purified Antibodies and Yeast Culture Supernatant. *J. Biomol. Screen.* **2016**, *21*, 88–95. [CrossRef]
17. Wang, Y.; Feng, P.; Sosic, Z.; Zang, L. Monitoring Glycosylation Profile and Protein Titer in Cell Culture Samples Using ZipChip CE-MS. *J. Anal. Bioanal. Technol.* **2017**, *8*. [CrossRef]
18. Pedersen, M.E.; Østergaard, J.; Jensen, H. In-Solution IgG Titer Determination in Fermentation Broth Using Affibodies and Flow-Induced Dispersion Analysis. *ACS Omega* **2020**, *5*, 10519–10524. [CrossRef] [PubMed]
19. Swartz, A.R.; Chen, W. Rapid Quantification of Monoclonal Antibody Titer in Cell Culture Harvests by Antibody-Induced Z-ELP-E2 Nanoparticle Cross-Linking. *Anal. Chem.* **2018**, *90*, 14447–14452. [CrossRef] [PubMed]
20. Chemmalil, L.; Prabhakar, T.; Kuang, J.; West, J.; Tan, Z.; Ehamparanathan, V.; Song, Y.; Xu, J.; Ding, J.; Li, Z. Online/at-line measurement, analysis and control of product titer and critical product quality attributes (CQAs) during process development. *Biotechnol. Bioeng.* **2020**. [CrossRef]
21. Willets, K.A.; Van Duyne, R.P. Localized Surface Plasmon Resonance Spectroscopy and Sensing. *Annu. Rev. Phys. Chem.* **2007**, *58*, 267–297. [CrossRef]
22. Bhagawati, M.; You, C.; Piehler, J. Quantitative Real-Time Imaging of Protein–Protein Interactions by LSPR Detection with Micropatterned Gold Nanoparticles. *Anal. Chem.* **2013**, *85*, 9564–9571. [CrossRef] [PubMed]
23. Liu, Y.; Zhang, N.; Li, P.; Yu, L.; Chen, S.; Zhang, Y.; Jing, Z.; Peng, W. Low-Cost Localized Surface Plasmon Resonance Biosensing Platform with a Response Enhancement for Protein Detection. *Nanomaterials* **2019**, *9*, 1019. [CrossRef] [PubMed]
24. Chavane, N.; Jacquemart, R.; Hoemann, C.D.; Jolicoeur, M.; De Crescenzo, G. At-line quantification of bioactive antibody in bioreactor by surface plasmon resonance using epitope detection. *Anal. Biochem.* **2008**, *378*, 158–165. [CrossRef] [PubMed]
25. Hampson, G.; Ward, T.H.; Cummings, J.; Bayne, M.; Tutt, A.; Cragg, M.S.; Dive, C.; Illidge, T.M. Validation of an ELISA for the determination of rituximab pharmacokinetics in clinical trials subjects. *J. Immunol. Methods* **2010**, *360*, 30–38. [CrossRef] [PubMed]
26. Liu, X.F.; Wang, X.; Weaver, R.J.; Calliste, L.; Xia, C.; He, Y.J.; Chen, L. Validation of a gyrolab™ assay for quantification of rituximab in human serum. *J. Pharmacol. Toxicol. Methods* **2012**, *65*, 107–114. [CrossRef]
27. Satzer, P.; Jungbauer, A. High-capacity protein A affinity chromatography for the fast quantification of antibodies: Two-wavelength detection expands linear range. *J. Sep. Sci.* **2018**, *41*, 1791–1797. [CrossRef]

Publisher's Note: MDPI stays neutral with regard to jurisdictional claims in published maps and institutional affiliations.

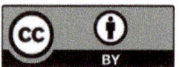

© 2020 by the authors. Licensee MDPI, Basel, Switzerland. This article is an open access article distributed under the terms and conditions of the Creative Commons Attribution (CC BY) license (http://creativecommons.org/licenses/by/4.0/).

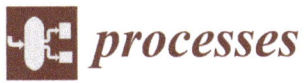

Article

Dielectric Spectroscopy to Improve the Production of rAAV Used in Gene Therapy

Daniel A. M. Pais [1,2,3], Chris Brown [3], Anastasia Neuman [3], Krishanu Mathur [3], Inês A. Isidro [1,2], Paula M. Alves [1,2] and Peter G. Slade [3,*]

1. iBET—Instituto de Biologia Experimental e Tecnológica, Apartado 12, 2781-901 Oeiras, Portugal; dpais@ibet.pt (D.A.M.P.); iaisidro@ibet.pt (I.A.I.); marques@ibet.pt (P.M.A.)
2. ITQB-NOVA, Instituto de Tecnologia Química e Biológica António Xavier, Universidade Nova de Lisboa, Av. da República, 2780-157 Oeiras, Portugal
3. Voyager Therapeutics, 75 Sidney St, Cambridge, MA 02139, USA; chrisb3c@gmail.com (C.B.); annaneu@seas.upenn.edu (A.N.); kmathur@vygr.com (K.M.)
* Correspondence: pslade@vygr.com

Received: 2 October 2020; Accepted: 10 November 2020; Published: 13 November 2020

Abstract: The insect cell-baculovirus expression vector system is an established method for large scale recombinant adeno-associated virus (rAAV) production, largely due to its scalability and high volumetric productivities. During rAAV production it is critical to monitor process parameters such as *Spodoptera frugiperda* (Sf9) cell concentration, infection timing, and cell harvest viabilities since they can have a significant influence on rAAV productivity and product quality. Herein we developed the use of dielectric spectroscopy as a process analytical technology (PAT) tool used to continuously monitor the production of rAAV in 2 L stirred tank bioreactors, achieving enhanced control over the production process. This study resulted in improved manufacturing robustness through continuous monitoring of cell culture parameters, eliminating sampling needs, increasing the accuracy of infection timing, and reliably estimating the time of harvest. To increase the accuracy of baculovirus infection timing, the cell growth/permittivity model was coupled to a feedback loop with real-time monitoring. This system was able to predict baculovirus infection timing up to 24 h in advance for greatly improved accuracy of infection and ensuring consistent high rAAV productivities. Furthermore, predictive models were developed based on the dielectric measurements of the culture. These multiple linear regression-based models resulted in correlation coefficients (Q^2) of 0.89 for viable cell concentration, 0.97 for viability, and 0.92 for cell diameter. Finally, models were developed to predict rAAV titer providing the capability to distinguish in real time between high and low titer production batches.

Keywords: AAV—adeno-associated virus; insect cell-baculovirus; gene therapy; cell culture monitoring; process analytical technology; dielectric spectroscopy

1. Introduction

Recombinant adeno-associated viruses (rAAV) are an ideal candidate gene therapy vector for many diseases, due to their ability to transduce nondividing cells from several tissues maintaining a long-term gene expression. rAAV also possess low immunogenicity compared to other viral vectors and are resilient to industry manufacturing methodologies, long-time storage, and in vivo administration [1,2].

While several biological systems have been adapted for rAAV production, the insect cell-baculovirus expression vector system (IC-BEVS) is very amenable for large scale rAAV production. Insect cells possess scalable and GMP-compatible characteristics, since they can grow in suspension to high cell densities in serum-free conditions [3]. As for the baculovirus, its use as a vector relies on the high recombinant protein production yields achieved and the absence of mammalian-derived products [4]. This combination resulted in several approved products, targeting Influenza (Flublok®), cancer (Cervarix® and Provenge®), and at least one rAAV-based gene therapy (Glybera™) [5,6]. Production of rAAV in the IC-BEVS requires two baculovirus: one coding for the AAV rep and cap functions and the other one providing the transgene flanked by the AAV Inverted Terminal Repeats (ITRs) [7].

Since 2004, with the introduction of the Process Analytical Technology (PAT) initiative by the USA Food and Drug administration (FDA) [8], regulatory entities have become increasingly more stringent regarding the end product quality attributes of biopharmaceutical products [9]. By encouraging the pharmaceutical industry to develop tools to characterize the pharmaceutical product and manufacturing process, in the end yielding biological products with consistent quality, the PAT initiative facilitates regulatory approval of new drugs. With that aim, the use of real-time monitoring tools for process characterization and product monitoring is strongly encouraged [9,10].

The ability to monitor in real-time the insect cell-baculovirus system would be greatly beneficial for manufacturing robustness particularly around the time of infection and the time of harvest. Infection timing and cell density have been shown to be critical parameters to maintain cell specific productivities (number of rAAV particles produced per cell and per unit time) [11,12]. Harvest timing also remains critical giving the lytic nature of the baculovirus and consequential release of proteases, which can compromise product quality [11,13–15]. Finally, the ability to estimate the rAAV titer in real-time is also highly desirable to harvest rAAV when its concentration is higher and as a means to monitor production batches.

Several types of sensors have been applied for monitoring of cell culture processes, based on imaging techniques [16–18] and spectroscopy such as infrared (mid and near), Raman, and fluorescence [15,19–22].

Another spectroscopy tool with proven applications for monitoring cell size and biovolume is dielectric spectroscopy, as demonstrated for bacteria, yeast, plant, and mammalian cells [22–27], with several authors reporting its application for monitoring insect cells in suspension [28–33]. This technique is based on the detection of the cell dielectric potential: when an electric field is applied to viable cells, they behave like small capacitors and polarize with a frequency-dependent response. This is due to the dielectric proprieties of the lipid based-cell membrane and the presence of conductive solutes in the extracellular medium and in the cytoplasm [34]. This charge can be detected and quantified, being reported as permittivity (capacitance per membrane area). As such, dielectric spectroscopy is ideal for monitoring infection-based processes, because of the effect that virus formation and release have on the cell membrane as well as in the intracellular composition of the cells [33,35].

The application of dielectric spectroscopy to monitor viral vector production processes is reported in several other works: Zeiser and coworkers correlated permittivity measurements with cell swelling due to intracellular baculovirus production [28]; Ansorge et al. followed the lentivirus budding process by monitoring physiological changes in infected producer cells [36]; Petiot et al. identified critical infection phases in enveloped and nonenveloped viruses, produced using transfection and infection methods [33]; Grein and coworkers used the culture permittivity measurements to detect the optimal harvest time in a oncolytic virus production process [13]; Negrete et al. correlated *Spodoptera frugiperda* (Sf9) cell diameter with rAAV production yield, decreasing the optimal harvest time by 24 h [31]. However, so far there is a lack solutions to monitor the accumulation of viral vectors in real-time [33], which was not addressed in the cited works.

Herein, we explored the capabilities of dielectric spectroscopy for use with the insect cell-baculovirus system during manufacturing of rAAV for gene therapy. To accurately predict baculovirus infection timing a feedback control strategy was developed using on-line permittivity values which greatly improved manufacturing robustness. Additionally, the ability of dielectric spectroscopy to monitor the cell physiological state was explored and prediction models were built for viable cell concentration, viability, and diameter. Finally, by combining the permittivity readings at

18 different frequencies with the beta-dispersion parameters determined for the system, we built a permittivity-based soft sensor for the estimation of intracellular rAAV titers in real-time.

2. Materials and Methods

2.1. Cell line and Culture Medium

Spodoptera frugiperda (Sf9) cells were routinely cultivated in 5 L Corning shake flasks with 3 L working volume of ESF-AF medium (Expression Systems™, Davis, CA, USA), at 27 °C with an agitation rate of 80 rpm in an Innova 44R incubator (orbital motion diameter = 2.54 cm, Eppendorf, Enfield, CT, USA). Cell concentration and viability were determined using a Vi-Cell XR Cell Counter (Beckman Coulter, Indianapolis, IN, USA).

2.2. Generation of Transgene-Bacmid and Rep/Cap-Bacmid

A transgene-bacmid and Rep/Cap-bacmid were generated according to a standard Tn7 transposition-based protocol, described as follows. A bacmid artificial chromosome (BAC) was used to generate the transgene-bacmid and Rep/Cap-bacmid, which includes the genome of *Autographa californica multicapsid nucleopolyhedrosis* virus along with an origin of replication that allows low-copy replication in *Escherichia coli* (*E. coli*). Briefly, donor plasmids including either the transgene or AAV rep/cap genes were delivered into DH10Bac™ *E. coli* by a standard heat-shock transformation. These *E. coli* cells contain the bacmid shuttle vector bMON14272 and helper plasmid pMON7124 that encodes the Tn7 transposase complex. Expression of the Tn7 transposase catalyzes excision of the nucleotides spanning (and including) the element Tn7L to the element Tn7R and insertion of these excised nucleotides into the mini-attTn7 site present in the bacmid shuttle vector bMON14272.

2.3. Generation of Transgene-BEV and Rep/Cap-BEV

The resulting transgene-bacmid and Rep/Cap-bacmid were purified. Sf9 cells were then transfected with either the transgene-bacmid or Rep/Cap-bacmid resulting in the expression of the baculovirus genes and the production of the infectious baculovirus expression vectors (BEVs): transgene-BEV or Rep/Cap-BEV, respectively. Briefly, a vial of Sf9 cells was thawed and suspended in protein free SFX Insect™ cell culture media and serially passaged at 26–28 °C until the viability was ≥80% and the diameter was 13–15 μm. This culture was used to prepare a cell suspension of approximately 1×10^6 cells/mL, which was seeded onto culture plates. Once the cells were attached to the plates, media was removed and replaced with a solution of Grace's medium (ThermoFisher Scientific, Waltham, MA, USA) and Cellfectin transfection reagent (ThermoFisher Scientific, Waltham, MA, USA) containing either the purified transgene-bacmid or Rep/Cap-bacmid. The transfected plates were incubated initially for 4–5 h. After removal of the transfection solution, fresh SFX Insect™ cell culture media was added, and the plate was incubated for an additional 3–4 days at 27 °C. The resulting BEVs were harvested, dispensed into a tube, and stored at 2–8 °C. Baculovirus titer was determined by using a BacPAK™ Baculovirus Rapid Titer Kit (Clontech Laboratories Inc. Mountain View, CA, USA or equivalent).

2.4. Generation of Rep/Cap- and Transgene-Baculovirus Infected Insect Cells (BIIC) Banks

Sf9 cells were expanded in shake flasks. Upon reaching the desired viable cell density and viability, the cells were infected with either the transgene-BEV or Rep/Cap-BEV at a multiplicity of infection of 0.01 and incubated for 48 ± 6 h, based on the protocol developed by Wasilko et al. [37]. The resulting Rep/Cap-BIICs and transgene-BIICs were pelleted by centrifugation, resuspended in 1× Cryopreservation medium which consists 1:1 (*v:v*) of SFX Insect™ cell culture media and 2× Cryopreservation medium (14% *v/v* DMSO, 11% *m/v* trehalose in SFX Insect™ cell culture media) and transferred into cryovials. The BIIC banks were frozen and stored at ≤−65 °C. The baculovirus titer was determined as described above.

2.5. Production of rAAV Using Rep/Cap-BIIC and Transgene-BIIC Coinfection

To produce rAAV in these experiments, the typical process would include a Sf9 growth phase of 3 days to a desired cell density, a baculovirus infection at a predetermined MOI, a baculovirus/rAAV expansion phase for 6 additional days and a harvest on day 9. Sf9 host cells were grown as a batch culture and coinfected with the two BIIC banks: Rep/Cap-BIIC and transgene-BIIC. Rep/Cap-BIIC provided the AAV2 Rep (replicase) and AAV1 Cap (capsid) genes to form capsids into which transgenes are packaged. The transgene-BIIC provided the transgene expression cassette containing a promoter region, the gene of interest, and the 5′ and 3′ ITRs. The transgene used in these experiments cannot be disclosed for confidentially reasons, but its identity was not relevant to these studies. Coinfection of Sf9 cultures with both BIIC banks was done either at a low cell density (3×10^6 cells/mL) or high cell density (5×10^6 cells/mL) depending on the experiments. To maintain a consistent multiplicity of infection (MOI), BIIC infection amounts were controlled by using a previously determined ratio of Sf9 cell culture volume to BIIC bank volume.

2.6. Infection of Sf9 Cells with Empty-BIIC Control

Sf9 cells were also infected with the empty-BIIC which was used as a control for model development. The empty-BIIC did not encode for any recombinant AAV or baculovirus transgene, while still allowing infectious baculovirus replication and consequent cytopathic effects. Infection conditions using the empty-BIIC were identical to the transgene or Rep/Cap-BIIC infection conditions, as described above.

2.7. Estimation of rAAV Titer by qPCR

Recombinant adeno-associated virus (rAAV) intracellular titer was measured using an in-house developed absolute quantification real-time PCR assay. Briefly, independent duplicates of each sample are incubated with DNAse (TekNova, Hollister, CA, USA) at 37 °C, in order to degrade extracellular DNA. Subsequently DNAse I is inactivated by addition of EDTA and followed by incubation with proteinase K (TekNova, Hollister, CA, USA) at 55 °C to degrade the rAAV capsids and release the encapsidated DNA. Proteinase K was deactivated by heating to 95 °C for 10 min. Digested material was subsequently diluted 40-fold in 10 mM Tris, pH 7.5. A 7-point, 10-fold serially diluted plasmid standard (in duplicate), containing the target sequence, was included on the 96-well dilution plate (VWR, Radnor, PA, USA) to allow for absolute quantification. On a separate 96-well lightcycler plate (Roche, Pleasanton, CA, USA) final 5-fold dilutions of both samples and plasmid standards were prepared in PCR mix (primer probes (IDT, Coralville, IA, USA) + mastermix (ThermoFisher Scientific, Waltham, MA, USA) each and the resulting final plate(s) were analyzed on a LightCycler 480 II Real-time PCR Thermocycler (Roche, Pleasanton, CA, USA). The PCR cycle profile consists of an initial polymerase activation step at 95 °C for 10 m, followed by 45 cycles consisting of a denaturation step at 95 °C for 10 s, an annealing step at 60 °C for 10 s, at the end of the 45 cycles a final extension step at 72 °C for 10 s was performed. Amplification results were analyzed using Roche Lightcycler 480 Software, samples and standards were indicated as appropriate and previously established plasmid standard values (copy numbers determined by orthogonal means) were entered. The software establishes a calibration curve and calculates reaction efficiency and standard curve error. If the curve passes preset acceptance criteria the samples are interpolated on the standard curve and the copy number for each sample is back-calculated using the total dilution factor.

2.8. Bioreactor Cultures and Sample Processing

Bioreactor cultures were performed in benchtop Finesse 3 L bioreactors (Finesse Solutions Inc, Santa Clara, CA, USA) with 1.6 L culture volume, equipped with one turbine with three blades tilted at 45° angle ("elephant ear" turbine). Temperature control (27 °C) was achieved using a heating jacket. Dissolved oxygen (DO) concentration was kept at 40% by continuous flow of air over the headspace and on-demand supply of air and O_2 mixtures using a L-shaped sparger in the bottom of the vessel.

The stirring rate was kept at 200 rpm. All controller action was ensured by Finesse Controllers and DeltaV software (St. Louis, MO, USA). Bioreactors were seeded at 1.1×10^6 Sf9 cells/mL. Infection was performed at different cell densities: 3×10^6 cells/mL for "standard", "empty" and "blend" batches and 5×10^6 cells/mL for "cell density effect" batches (see Figure 1), at the volume of culture to BIIC volume ratios indicated above. "Empty" and "blend" batches were added to increase model robustness and decouple permittivity signals associated to rAAV production from permittivity signals induced by Sf9 cell growth and baculovirus replication. For empty runs, empty-BIICs were added to the Sf9 cultures at a total volume to volume ratio as both the Rep/Cap and transgene-BIICs. For "blend" batches, both "standard" and "empty" infections were performed in separate bioreactors. On day 2 post-infection, cells from both reactors were transferred to another bioreactor, with the following ratios of "standard" to "empty" (100:0; 65:35; 40:60; 10:90), in a total of 1.3 L working volume. The multiplicity of infection (MOI) was kept constant for every batch.

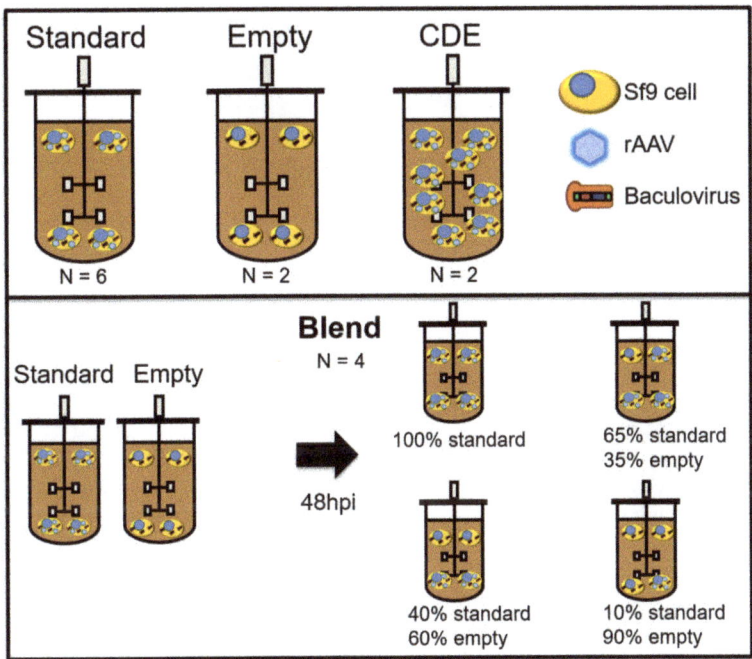

Figure 1. Overview of the different batches used for model calibration. "Standard" runs represent a normal infection process, with coinfection with Rep/Cap and transgene-BIICs (baculovirus-infected insect cells). "Empty" runs were infected with an empty-BIIC, a BIIC which was infected with a baculovirus vector devoid of any transgene, but still able to replicate and induce cytopathic effects in infected cells. Cell density effect (CDE) runs are like "standard" runs, except that infection was performed at 5×10^6 cells/mL instead of 3×10^6. "Blend" runs started with separate "standard" and "empty" batches. Two days after infection, cells from both reactors were transferred to new bioreactors, with the indicated proportions of each batch. Hpi—hours post-infection.

The Incyte sensor (Hamilton, Reno, NV, USA) was inserted in a standard 19 mm bioreactor top port, to perform in situ permittivity and conductivity measurements. After sterilization, sensor readings were zeroed with culture medium, after allowing enough time for the permittivity and conductivity signals to stabilize at 27 °C. Permittivity and conductivity measurements were performed every 6 min, with permittivity measurements obtained in a range of 18 frequencies between 300 and

10,000 kHz. Measurements were recorded using the ArcView instrument (Hamilton, Reno, NV, USA). In the "blend" experiments, only the "blend" bioreactors were monitored with Incyte, this being the reason why there are no permittivity measurements before day 2 post-infection.

Sampling for determination of reference variables was done three times per day before infection and four times per day after infection. At each sampling point, cell concentration and viability were measured using Vi-cell Counter. For rAAV determination, 10 mL of culture supernatant were subjected to a clarification step (1000 g, 10 min) to separate intra and extracellular rAAV. Supernatant was discarded, and the pellet resuspended in an equal volume of fresh medium, to which a 1.3 mL of lysis solution was added. Samples were left agitating at 27 °C, 200 rpm, for approximately 24 h, centrifuged (4000× g, 5 min), filtered through a 0.2 µm syringe filter and stored at 4 °C until analysis.

2.9. Process-to-Target Script to Predict Time of Infection

The process-to-target is an in-house script which runs in the JMP (SAS Institute, Cary, NC, USA) programming language. The process-to-target script predicts the infection timing based on all the measured permittivity values for the 1000 kHz frequency, considering timepoints from cell seeding to the moment the script is run. It is based in a time-weighted linear model of permittivity. Briefly, the script plots the permittivity values from the Incyte probe and the corresponding time in hours since the beginning of the run. Each data point is given a weight (Time^7), with later timepoints having a significantly higher weight when compared to earlier time points, avoiding the inherent nonlinearity of the initial portion of the permittivity curve (corresponding to the lag phase). A weighted linear model is then fit to the data and the model values are saved. Using the target permittivity, the model values are used to calculate the time in hours at which the culture will reach infection density. The time remaining to infection is also calculated using the current time. The script outputs the graphical results as demonstrated in Section 3.

2.10. Modeling Strategy and Software

A total of 14 bioreactors were run in different conditions: six "standard" runs, two "cell density effect" runs, two "empty" runs, and four "blend" runs (Figure 1). All analysis and modeling were performed in JMP v14 (SAS institute, Cary, NC, USA). The Incyte data consisted of 22 variables: permittivity measured at 18 different frequencies, medium conductivity and three beta-dispersion curve parameters (alpha, characteristic frequency, and Δε). All these variables were automatically calculated by the Incyte sensor. After run completion, the Incyte data was smoothed using a 30-min (five datapoints) moving average filter. This data was time-aligned with the corresponding sampling points (reference data). *Biovolume* was calculated based on the viable cell concentration and the cell diameter measurements, considering cells as perfect spheres (Equation (1)).

$$Biovolume = \text{Viable cell concentration} \times \frac{4}{3}\pi (cell\ radius)^3 \quad (1)$$

For calibrating the models, the offline reference data obtained from Vi-cell measurements and corresponding online averages for permittivity measurements were used. The dataset was divided into calibration and testing set, with two "standard" batches (numbered 5 and 7) as the testing set and the remaining belonging to the calibration set.

Models were developed using JMP "Fit model" platform. Briefly the 22 parameters were subjected to forward and backwards stepwise regression to find the most significant parameters to each of the reference variables. In the forward stepwise regression method, the most significant attribute was identified and added to the model, followed by identification and inclusion in the model of the second most significant attribute and so on. In a backwards stepwise regression method, all parameters were added to the model in the beginning and were stepwise removed according to their lack of significance to the model. The significance level considered was p-value = 0.05. For the most significant attributes, their two-level interactions and quadratics were also considered, using the same combination of forward and backwards stepwise regression.

RMSEs for calibration (RMSEC) and testing (RMSET) were calculated for all models (Equation (2)). The correlation coefficients of calibration and testing were calculated according to Equation (3) using calibration (R^2) or testing (Q^2) data.

In Equations (2) and (3), $\hat{y}$ represents a vector of model-predicted values and y represents the corresponding reference data; ncal and ntest represent the number of samples in the calibration or testing set, respectively. σ^2 represents sample variance.

$$RMSEC = \sqrt{\frac{\sum_{i=1}^{ncal}(\hat{y}-y)^2}{ncal}}. \quad RMSET = \sqrt{\frac{\sum_{i=1}^{nval}(\hat{y}-y)^2}{ntest}}. \quad (2)$$

$$R^2 = 1 - \frac{RMSEC^2}{\sigma^2}. \quad Q^2 = 1 - \frac{RMSET^2}{\sigma^2}. \quad (3)$$

3. Results

3.1. Accurate Prediction of Infection Timing Using Continuous Permittivity Monitoring

Accurate targeting of cell concentration at the time of baculovirus infection is critical to maintain rAAV titers due to the so called "cell density effect" [12]. To understand this critical parameter, Sf9 cells were infected with baculovirus expressing rAAV at different cell concentrations from 2×10^6 to 6×10^6 cell/mL. Figure 2A shows 3×10^6 cells/mL to be the ideal cell concentration at infection to reach a maximum titer value ($\approx 6 \times 10^{11}$ vg/mL). Infections above 3.5×10^6 cells/mL demonstrated a dramatic decrease in rAAV titer and cell specific productivity. At 5–6 $\times 10^6$ cell/mL rAAV titers were below the limit of detection. Figure 2B shows the linear relationship between specific rAAV productivity and Sf9 concentration at infection.

To better understand cell concentration variability at time of infection, growth data from multiple 2 L bioreactor production runs were analyzed. Figure 2C shows significant batch to batch variability in cell growth, most likely due to small changes in inoculation density. For example, if the target cell concentration at infection to reach maximum rAAV titer was 3×10^6 cells/mL, the timing of infection would vary anywhere from 45 to 65 h post inoculation, which necessitates constant sampling close to the time of infection in order to achieve an accurate cell concentration.

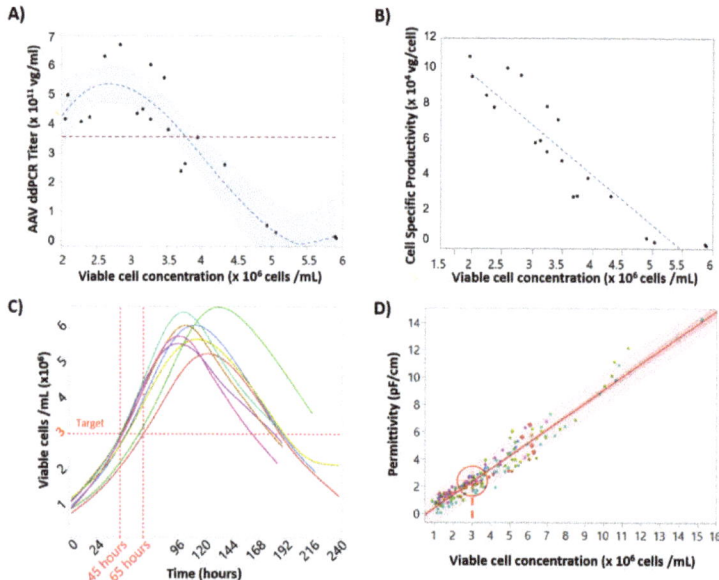

Figure 2. Impact of cell concentration on recombinant adeno-associated virus (rAAV) titers and correlations between cell concentration, cell specific productivity, and permittivity. (**A**) Model (dashed line) and 95% confidence intervals (shaded area) for the relationship between rAAV titer at day 6 and cell concentration at infection. (**B**) Linear correlation between cell concentration at infection and rAAV specific productivity. (**C**) Viable cell concentration time-course profiles for the "standard" batches, with coinfection with Rep/Cap and transgene-BIICs (baculovirus-infected insect cells). The time when the cells reached the target cell concentration at infection can vary up to 24 h. (**D**) Correlation between viable cell concentration measured by Vi-cell and permittivity values measured by the Incyte sensor. The target value of viable cell concentration of 3×10^6 cells/mL is represented by a target, corresponding to a permittivity value of 2.2 pF/cm (95% confidence interval = 2.18–2.34 pF/cm). $R^2_{adjs} = 0.94$.

To make infection timing robust and operator-independent, a strategy of predicting the time of infection was developed called process-to-target. This strategy was based on the real-time availability of permittivity measurements provided by the Incyte sensor. The first step was to determine the correlation between permittivity and viable cell concentration, which is linear during the exponential growth stage, as shown in Figure 2D. As such, the permittivity corresponding to the target cell concentration was determined to be 2.2 pF/cm (95% confidence intervals (CI) of 2.18–2.34 pF/cm). The process-to-target script was then developed to continuously predict the timing of infection in real-time after each permittivity measurement, where the model inputs were permittivity, acquisition time, and the target permittivity value. To obtain a linear model from a nonlinear dataset, the process to target model used a weighted fit where a weighted time was calculated by giving more weight to later time points. As expected, this linear model demonstrated poor prediction accuracy at early time points but as the cell growth progressed these model predictions would converge on a time at which the permittivity would reach the target of 2.2 pF/cm with an accurate prediction occurring 24–48 h in advance. This is demonstrated in Figure 3, where an accurate prediction for baculovirus infection was achieved at 24 h post inoculation, providing >24 h in advance warning of the infection time.

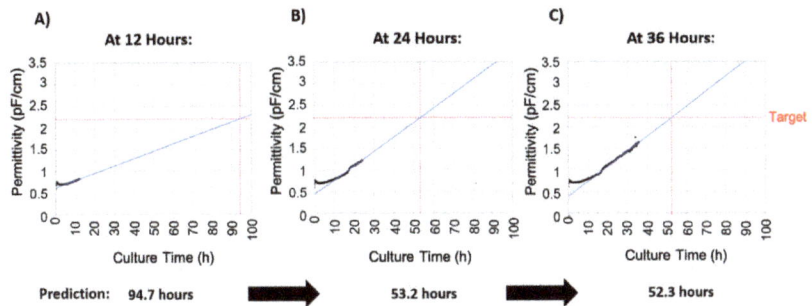

Figure 3. Outputs of the process-to-target. The script was run at different times after inoculation, and the infection timing predictions are indicated below each image. For this figure, batch 5 was used, in which the target was reached at 50.8 h. Permittivity data is represented in black, the blue line represents model predictions, and the red lines are the target (vertical axis) and the predicted time the target will be reached (horizontal axis). (**A**) Process-to-target script run 12 h after seeding. (**B**) Process-to-target script run 24 h after seeding. (**C**) Process-to-target script run 36 h after seeding.

To validate "process to target" predictions, the algorithm was tested on 10 2-L bioreactor runs. Table 1 shows the actual vs. the predicted infection timings at 6, 12, 24, and 48 h post-inoculation. As stated, prediction accuracy improved at later time points as the availability of more data allowed the model to converge on the actual time. Accurate predictions were obtained as early as 24 h post-inoculation in all runs and the process-to-target strategy clearly demonstrated a robust method to ensure accuracy of a critical process parameter were the manufacturing operator can be informed well in advance the precise time of baculovirus infection.

Table 1. Application of the process-to-target script to each of 10 batches monitored using the Incyte probe at several process timepoints after seeding. The numbers in the prediction columns represent the predicted infection time (in hours post-seeding). Actual time indicates the time in hours that the permittivity equaled the nominal target of 2.2 pF/cm. "N/A" indicates a timepoint that was past the point where the target was reached. For the details on batch nomenclature, the reader is referred to Figure 1. CDE = cell density effect. The data presented in this table was calculated after batch completion.

Batch Number	Batch Type	Prediction				Actual Time (h)
		6 h	12 h	24 h	48 h	
1	Standard	−648	129	53	54	55
2	Standard	−299	73	59	59	59
3	Empty	458	95	64	53	52
4	Standard	196	114	59	56	55
5	Standard	213	95	53	50	51
6	Standard	136	56	37	N/A	36
7	Standard	−92	108	53	57	52
8	CDE	−120	156	65	65	61
9	Empty	−746	112	50	N/A	48
10	CDE	553	107	56	55	54

3.2. Dielectric Spectroscopy for Monitoring the Progress of Baculovirus Infection In Situ

Correlation of the dielectric spectroscopy parameters conductivity, permittivity, beta-dispersion, and characteristic frequency to critical process parameters such as cell concentration, cell viability, and virus production allows for the development of on-line models to monitor critical process parameters. As shown in Figure 4A, culture conductivity increases simultaneously with the onset of baculovirus-induced cell lysis, suggesting that conductivity can be used to build predictive models of cell death post viral infection (Figure S1). The beta-dispersion curve and curve parameters (Δε, α, and characteristic frequency) can be derived from measurements of permittivity over a wide range (Figure 4B). This curve is indicative of changes in the cell state during the production process [33] and can be used to understand changes in cell size and viability (Figure S2). Permittivity has been shown to correspond to cell concentration [32,33] and can be used to calculate a biomass or cell density (Figure 4C). The characteristic frequency signal has been used to monitor baculovirus budding from infected cells, through a "v-shape" profile in the characteristic frequency of the culture [33]. In Figure 4D we also demonstrate this "v-shaped" profile in the infected cells. This way, dielectric spectroscopy is ideally suited to follow in real-time a complete insect cell baculovirus infection process: cell seeding, cell growth, infection density, baculovirus-induced cell diameter increase, cell growth arrest, and finally cell death.

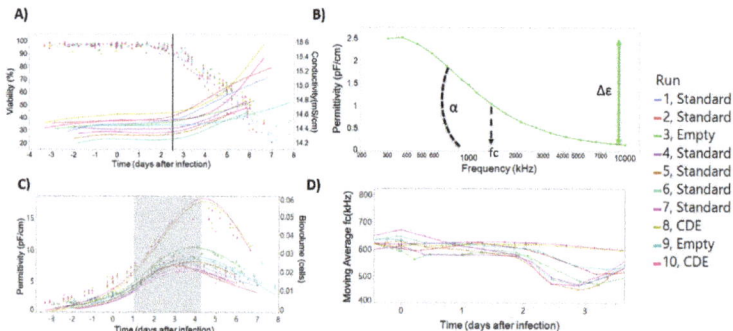

Figure 4. Incyte measurements can be correlated with the progress of baculovirus infection in insect cells. (**A**) The onset of baculovirus-induced cell lysis (viability, represented with circles) can be detected by the simultaneous onset of conductivity increase (smooth lines, measured by Incyte). (**B**) Beta-dispersion curve 24 h after seeding, for batch number 1. The beta-dispersion allows calculation of variables such as Δε, α, and characteristic frequency, which are indicative of the cell state during the infection process. (**C**) Visual inspection of the permittivity profile allows to follow the three phases of the production process (separated by the shaded area): cell growth, cell diameter increase due to baculovirus infection, and baculovirus-induced cell lysis. Circles represent biovolume calculations based on the measured diameter and considering cells as perfect spheres, and smooth lines the Incyte permittivity measurements at 1000 kHz. (**D**) The characteristic frequency (frequency corresponding to the beta-dispersion curve inflection point) time profile is shown. The "v-shaped" profile after 2 days post infection has been postulated to be correlated with baculovirus release from cells elsewhere [33].

Prediction models for viable cell concentration, percent viability, and average cell diameter were built using the above dielectric spectroscopy parameters and the calibration/testing sets described in Section 2. Figure 5A shows the observed vs. predicted values for the viable cell concentration model, giving an R^2 value of 0.96. To validate the model, time-course profiles of viable cell concentration measured by Vi-Cell for two batches were compared with the corresponding model predictions (Figure 5B). The models demonstrated high accuracy with a Q^2 of 0.89 and only a slight underestimation of the viable cell concentration.

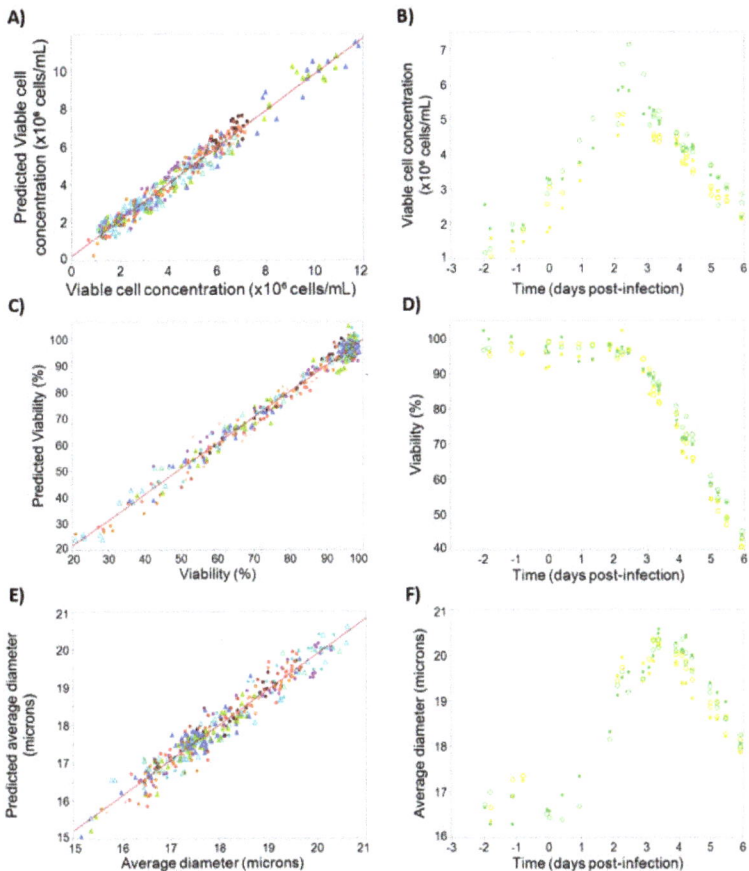

Figure 5. Calibration and testing data for viable cell concentration, viability, and average cell diameter. On the left, observed and predicted values for the calibration dataset, for (**A**) viable cell concentration, $R^2 = 0.96$; (**C**) viability, $R^2 = 0.98$; (**E**) diameter, $R^2 = 0.94$. Batches are represented by different colors, with filled triangles representing "cell density effect" batches, empty triangles representing "empty" batches, and filled circles representing "standard" and "blend" batches. On the right, time-course profiles for the testing set, for (**B**) viable cell concentration, $Q^2 = 0.89$; (**D**) viability ($Q^2 = 0.97$); (**F**) diameter ($Q^2 = 0.92$). Batches are represented by different colors, with reference data shown as open circles and corresponding model-predicted values shown as filled circles.

For percent viability models the observed vs. predicted profile can be seen in Figure 5C, giving an R^2 of 0.98 with a large dynamic range. The prediction profiles (Figure 5D) are also remarkably accurate with Q^2 of 0.98. This prediction accuracy held throughout growth phase, stationary phase, and death phase, demonstrating the prediction model can be used throughout culture. Finally, since measuring changes in cell diameter is often a useful indicator of the progress of baculovirus infection, models for cell diameter were developed giving an R^2 of 0.94 and a high validation accuracy with Q^2 of 0.92 (Figure 5E,F). Similar to the viability models, cell diameter models were accurate during all phases of the cell growth and infection.

3.3. Detection of rAAV-Induced Signals Using Multiple Linear Regression

A prediction model to measure in real-time intracellular rAAV production was developed using similar modeling strategies to the process parameter models. Supernatant rAAV concentrations were not considered since dielectric spectroscopy measures variations in the intracellular composition of the cell. The model was trained using a bioreactor dataset shown in Figure 6 where both the intracellular rAAV titer (rAAV quantified in the lysed pellet solution) and the specific rAAV titer are shown (intracellular titer normalized by viable cell concentration). As described in Section 2, rAAV production was decoupled from cell growth and baculovirus replication by adjusting infection cell densities and using a "blend batch" strategy (Figure 1). This resulted in a dataset giving a wide range of rAAV titers at both low and high cell concentrations. In particular, specific rAAV production titer was greatly reduced by infecting cells at high cell density (Figure 6B, blue and green triangles), where infection at a low cell density gave much higher titers (filled circles). The "blend batch" strategy also had the desired effect of providing rAAV concentration profiles at different ranges and is shown as the open circles in Figure 6.

Using this dataset, a multiple linear regression model to predict rAAV by dielectric spectroscopy was developed. The observed vs. predicted dataset used for the model calibration gave an R^2 of 0.71 (Figure 7A). Good predictions were obtained for blend batches, which confirmed the model ability to predict rAAV production batches. The model was validated using two independent bioreactor runs as a testing set, resulting in acceptable predictions with a Q^2 of 0.77 (Figure 7B).

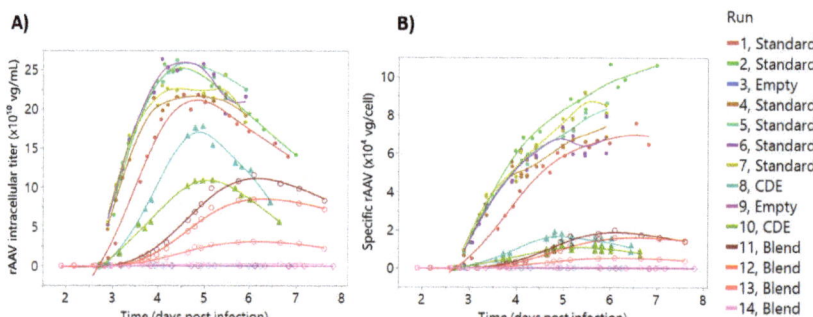

Figure 6. Recombinant adeno-associated virus (rAAV) intracellular production profiles. The datapoints represent vector genome quantification. Filled circles represent "standard" batches, triangles represent "cell density effect" batches, empty diamonds represent "empty batches", and the empty circles represent "blend batches". For the details on batch nomenclature, the reader is referred to Figure 1. Lines represent a smooth of the reference data, unrelated with model predictions. (**A**) rAAV intracellular titer, the rAAV concentration after lysing pellet from 10 mL of culture. (**B**) Specific rAAV titer. Same data as (**A**) normalized by the number of viable cells at the corresponding sampling time.

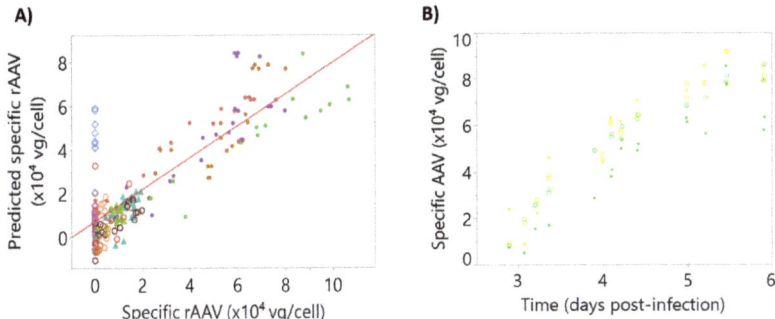

Figure 7. Calibration and testing data for intracellular specific recombinant adeno-associated virus (rAAV). Batches are represented by different colors. (**A**) Observed and predicted values for the dataset used for model calibration, $R^2 = 0.71$. Batches are represented by different colors, with filled triangles representing "cell density effect" batches, empty diamonds representing "empty" batches, filled circles representing "standard" batches, and empty circles representing "blend" batches. (**B**) Intracellular specific rAAV time-course profiles for the testing set, $Q^2 = 0.77$. Reference data is represented by open circles and corresponding model-predicted values are shown as filled circles.

4. Discussion

In this work we employed dielectric spectroscopy for accurate prediction of infection timing in the insect cell-baculovirus system. Moreover, we developed predictive models for cell concentration, viability, diameter, and rAAV production, which can be used to follow the progress of baculovirus infection and recombinant AAV production in real-time.

The time of infection is one of the most important process parameters in the insect cell system, with direct implications on rAAV production [11,34]. Current methods for infection timing require frequent offline cell-counting and are prone to error due to equipment variability and operator dependency. Additionally, frequent sampling increases the chance for contamination. Real-time, continuous monitoring of viable cell concentration can alleviate this issue. One of the real-time monitoring tools extensively applied to monitor cell concentration in cell culture processes is dielectric spectroscopy [14,22,38], which has also been demonstrated in the insect-cell system [28–33]. Taking advantage of the frequent Incyte permittivity measurements and the high correlation between permittivity and cell concentration (Figure 2D), we applied dielectric spectroscopy to predict infection timing (Figure 3). An in-house JMP script (process-to-target) was developed, which used real-time permittivity data to accurately predict infection timing. The prediction model was designed to converge on an accurate prediction of infection timing as more data became available (Table 1). This tool was able to predict infection timing within 10% of the actual infection time as early as 24 h post-inoculation and at least 24 h pre-infection. This amount of prior notice would allow for more robust manufacturing and batch to batch consistency. Importantly, the process-to-target script was operator independent, reducing dependence on sampling and any potential operator error at one of the most critical stages of the rAAV production process.

The process-to-target relies on the linear correlations between permittivity and cell concentration and viability and conductivity (Figure S3). However, the correlations obtained for one batch cannot be used directly in another batch. We even detected a significant difference in the obtained linear regression slope for permittivity and cell concentration in different cell banks (results not shown). Moreover, even though the same medium was used in parallel bioreactors and the Incyte probe was zeroed in the medium, the conductivity measurements had a baseline reading which is different between batches (Figure 4A). Therefore, the process-to-target was developed as a feedback loop that continually adjusted its prediction in real-time making it sufficiently robust for batch to batch manufacturing purposes.

Further development of the process-to-target script is ongoing. Taking into account the inverse linear correlation between the onset of viability decrease and the onset of conductivity increase (Figure 4A and Figure S1), experiments are continuing to switch from a "by day" -based harvest into a viability-based harvest and adapting the process-to-target to the conductivity measurements to accurately predict harvest time. The choice of the best viability to harvest is dependent not only on the final rAAV titer but also the vector potency and the overall downstream yield [11,13,14].

Due to the batch to batch variability, robust prediction models for viable cell density, viability, cell diameter, and rAAV titer based on conductivity and/or permittivity-only measurements could not be used. Consequently, the beta-dispersion curve was included in modeling these critical process variables which reduced any variability seen in the datasets and improved model robustness. These changes can be quantified by calculating the beta-dispersion curve parameters over time: the difference between the low and high frequency plateaus ($\Delta\varepsilon$), the Cole-Cole α (α), and the curve inflexion point (characteristic frequency, fc). These parameters have been shown to be useful for characterizing the culture and building accurate models. For instance, α is related with the distribution of the dielectric properties in the population and the cell shape and size [32,39]; $\Delta\varepsilon$ is proportional to cell concentration and biovolume [33], and fc has been demonstrated to be correlated with the cell death phase and virus budding [33,36]. A more in-depth review of the biological meaning of each parameter can be seen in Dabros et al. [39].

The models for viable cell concentration, viability, cell diameter, and rAAV titer are shown in Figures 5 and 7. They were built using the previously described calibration datasets and the above-mentioned beta-dispersion parameters and frequency measurements. Besides multiple linear regression, we also tested partial least squares (PLS) regression and artificial neural networks. Multiple linear regression models combined simplicity with accurate predictions, and thus it was the strategy followed for developing predictive models. The high Q^2 obtained for each model demonstrated that dielectric spectroscopy signals can be used to predict these critical process parameters.

For the development of rAAV titer models (Figure 7) extracellular rAAV titer was excluded from the models because our hypothesis was that most rAAV-induced alterations to the cell state would be detected through variations in the intracellular composition of the cell. Moreover, measuring intracellular rAAV data contributed to an increased understanding of our production process (Figure 6). For instance, as culture progresses and cell lysis starts to occur, the number of viable cells producing rAAV decreases (Figure 6). Due to this decreasing number of viable cells, the rAAV production tends to plateau around day 5. As such, we may be able to harvest our process one day earlier, depending on rAAV product quality profiles. The addition of cultures infected at higher cell density was intended to introduce variability in the model, based on the known drop in cell specific productivities when infecting high cell density cultures [40–42]. Similarly, the "blend" batch strategy was intended to decouple rAAV permittivity signals from cell and baculovirus-induced permittivity changes. This strategy was successful in generating batches with decreasing rAAV concentration, keeping the cell concentration and baculovirus infection at similar levels (Figure 6). However, even though infection was performed at 3×10^6 cells/mL, these runs have a rAAV production profile similar to the "cell density effect" batches (Figure S4). This was likely associated to the stressful condition of transferring the cells from the first bioreactor to the "blend" bioreactor. Although the "blend" strategy produced titers lower than expected, the resulting calibration set was more than sufficient to develop an accurate model and did not impact model predictions.

Dielectric spectroscopy has previously been used to monitor baculovirus release from infected cells. Petiot and coworkers found a characteristic "V-shape" profile in the characteristic frequency time-course profile, and associated that signal with viral budding from the infected cells [33]. In Figure 4D, we also observed a significant drop in the permittivity around day 2 post-infection. Given that our infection process takes place at a very low MOI, it takes 2 days to infect a significant proportion of the Sf9 population for the baculovirus release from the cells be detectable. As a control group, the two "cell density effect" batches do not show the decrease in the characteristic frequency value on day 2, but instead on day 4, since the higher cell concentration at infection is able to delay detection of the cell growth arrest induced by baculovirus. Moreover, we were able to develop good prediction models for the cell diameter, an indicator of the progress of baculovirus infection [43,44]. This knowledge coupled to "V-shape" in characteristic frequency may be useful for characterizing the baculovirus release kinetics and prediction of baculovirus release from infected cells.

5. Conclusions

The work developed clearly shows dielectric spectroscopy can be used as a PAT tool for this system, not only by allowing accurate infection time determination, but also for rAAV production monitoring. The ability to estimate the time of infection more than 24 h before is invaluable for GMP settings, proving the usefulness of the process-to-target approach. The predictive models developed for critical process parameters demonstrate accurate predictions for viable cell concentration, viability, and diameter in an independent testing set, validating the chosen strategy, and can be used for developing viability-based harvest methods. The determined intracellular rAAV production profiles, together with the developed rAAV prediction models, allow to increase process knowledge regarding this process, and to possibly unveil new factors influencing rAAV production by conducting process alterations and supplements administration and assess their impact on rAAV production in real-time. Future studies will address the possibility of applying this tool for determination of rAAV quality characteristics, such as potency or ratio of empty to full particles.

Supplementary Materials: The following are available online at http://www.mdpi.com/2227-9717/8/11/1456/s1, Figure S1: Viability reference data and corresponding predictions using only the conductivity data, Figure S2: Representative beta dispersion curve evolution profiles for different culture phases, Figure S3: Linear correlation between permittivity and viable cell concentration and conductivity and viability, Figure S4: Scores for the two first principal components for all runs.

Author Contributions: Conceptualization, D.A.M.P. and P.G.S.; methodology, D.A.M.P., C.B., A.N., K.M., P.G.S.; software, C.B.; formal analysis, D.A.M.P., C.B., A.N., K.M., P.G.S.; investigation, D.A.M.P., A.N.; resources, P.G.S.; data curation, C.B.; writing—original draft preparation, D.A.M.P.; writing—review and editing, D.A.M.P., C.B., A.N., K.M., I.A.I., P.M.A., P.G.S.; visualization, D.A.M.P., I.A.I., P.M.A., P.G.S.; supervision, K.M., I.A.I., P.M.A., P.G.S.; project administration, P.G.S.; funding acquisition, P.G.S. All authors have read and agreed to the published version of the manuscript.

Funding: This research received no external funding.

Acknowledgments: The authors would like to thank Luís Maranga for his continual support of this research as well as the process development analytical team at Voyager for processing so many titer samples and the Cell Culture Development group for their support and help in setting up, running, and sampling reactors. Jacob Crowe from Hamilton is acknowledged for the initial set up of the system and exploratory data analysis. Finally, we would like to thank Tom Little of Thomas Little Consulting for his advice building JMP models and help in developing the process-to-target script.

Conflicts of Interest: Krishanu Mathur and Peter Slade are employees of Voyager Therapeutics, Inc. Chris Brown is employee of Vedere Bio. The remaining authors declare no conflict of interest. The founding sponsors had no role in the design of the study; in the collection, analyses, or interpretation of data; in the writing of the manuscript, and in the decision to publish the results.

Abbreviations

AAV	Adeno-associated virus
BEV	Baculovirus expression vector
BIIC	Baculovirus-infected insect cell
FDA	Food and Drug administration
ITR	Inverted Terminal Repeat
PAT	Process analytical technology
Sf9	*Spodoptera frugiperda* cell line

References

1. Xu, Z.; Shi, C.; Qian, Q. Scalable manufacturing methodologies for improving adeno-associated virus-based pharmaprojects. *Chin. Sci. Bull.* **2014**, *59*, 1845–1855. [CrossRef]
2. Galibert, L.; Merten, O.W. Latest developments in the large-scale production of adeno-associated virus vectors in insect cells toward the treatment of neuromuscular diseases. *J. Invertebr. Pathol.* **2011**, *107*, S80–S93. [CrossRef] [PubMed]
3. Penaud-Budloo, M.; LeComte, E.; Guy-Duché, A.; Saleun, S.; Roulet, A.; Lopez-Roques, C.; Tournaire, B.; Cogné, B.; Léger, A.; Blouin, V.; et al. Accurate Identification and Quantification of DNA Species by Next-Generation Sequencing in Adeno-Associated Viral Vectors Produced in Insect Cells. *Hum. Gene Ther. Methods* **2017**, *28*, 148–162. [CrossRef]
4. Yee, C.M.; Zak, A.J.; Hill, B.D.; Wen, F. The Coming Age of Insect Cells for Manufacturing and Development of Protein Therapeutics. *Ind. Eng. Chem. Res.* **2018**, *57*, 10061–10070. [CrossRef] [PubMed]
5. Monteiro, F. Rational Design of Insect Cell-based Vaccine Production—Bridging Metabolomics with Mathematical Tools to Study Virus-Host Interactions. Ph.D. Thesis, Instituto de Tecnologia Química e Biológica António Xavier, Universidade Nova de Lisboa, Oeiras, Portugal, September 2015.
6. Shahryari, A.; Jazi, M.S.; Mohammadi, S.; Nikoo, H.R.; Nazari, Z.; Hosseini, E.S.; Burtscher, I.; Mowla, S.J.; Lickert, H. Development and Clinical Translation of Approved Gene Therapy Products for Genetic Disorders. *Front. Genet.* **2019**, *10*, 868. [CrossRef] [PubMed]
7. Smith, R.H.; Levy, J.R.; Kotin, R.M. A Simplified Baculovirus-AAV Expression Vector System Coupled With One-step Affinity Purification Yields High-titer rAAV Stocks From Insect Cells. *Mol. Ther.* **2009**, *17*, 1888–1896. [CrossRef]
8. US Department of Health and Human Services; Food and Drug Administration (FDA); Center for Drug Evaluation and Research (CDER); Center for Veterinary Medicine (CVM); Office of Regulatory Affairs (ORA). Guidance for Industry PAT—A Framework for Innovative Pharmaceutical Development, Manufacturing and Quality Assurance Pharmaceutical CGMPs. 2004. Available online: https://www.fda.gov/media/71012/download (accessed on 20 March 2020).
9. Pais, D.A.; Carrondo, M.J.T.; Alves, P.M.; Teixeira, A.P. Towards real-time monitoring of therapeutic protein quality in mammalian cell processes. *Curr. Opin. Biotechnol.* **2014**, *30*, 161–167. [CrossRef]
10. Guerra, A.; Von Stosch, M.; Glassey, J. Toward biotherapeutic product real-time quality monitoring. *Crit. Rev. Biotechnol.* **2019**, *39*, 289–305. [CrossRef]
11. Lecina, M.; Soley, A.; Gracia, J.; Espunya, E.; Lazaro, B.; Cairó, J.; Gòdia, F. Application of on-line OUR measurements to detect actions points to improve baculovirus-insect cell cultures in bioreactors. *J. Biotechnol.* **2006**, *125*, 385–394. [CrossRef]
12. Estrada-Mondaca, S.; Ramirez, O.; Palomares, L. Principles and Applications of the Insect Cell-Baculovirus Expression Vector System. *Isol. Purif. Proteins* **2005**, *18*, 627–692.
13. Grein, T.A.; Loewe, D.; Dieken, H.; Salzig, D.; Weidner, T.; Czermak, P. High titer oncolytic measles virus production process by integration of dielectric spectroscopy as online monitoring system. *Biotechnol. Bioeng.* **2018**, *115*, 1186–1194. [CrossRef] [PubMed]
14. Nikolay, A.; Léon, A.; Schwamborn, K.; Genzel, Y.; Reichl, U. Process intensification of EB66® cell cultivations leads to high-yield yellow fever and Zika virus production. *Appl. Microbiol. Biotechnol.* **2018**, *102*, 8725–8737. [CrossRef] [PubMed]
15. Pais, D.A.M.; Portela, R.M.C.; Carrondo, M.J.T.; Isidro, I.A.; Alves, P.M. Enabling PAT in insect cell bioprocesses: In situ monitoring of recombinant adeno-associated virus production by fluorescence spectroscopy. *Biotechnol. Bioeng.* **2019**, *116*, 2803–2814. [CrossRef] [PubMed]
16. Loutfi, H.; Pellen, F.; Le Jeune, B.; Lteif, R.; Kallassy, M.; Le Brun, G.; Abboud, M. Real-time monitoring of bacterial growth kinetics in suspensions using laser speckle imaging. *Sci. Rep.* **2020**, *10*, 1–10. [CrossRef]
17. Janicke, B.; Kårsnäs, A.; Egelberg, P.; Alm, K. Label-free high temporal resolution assessment of cell proliferation using digital holographic microscopy. *Cytom. Part A* **2017**, *91*, 460–469. [CrossRef]
18. Pais, D.A.M.; Galrão, P.R.S.; Kryzhanska, A.; Barbau, J.; Isidro, I.A.; Alves, P.M. Holographic Imaging of Insect Cell Cultures: Online Non-Invasive Monitoring of Adeno-Associated Virus Production and Cell Concentration. *Processes* **2020**, *8*, 487. [CrossRef]

19. Qiu, J.; Arnold, M.A.; Murhammer, D.W. On-line near infrared bioreactor monitoring of cell density and concentrations of glucose and lactate during insect cell cultivation. *J. Biotechnol.* **2014**, *173*, 106–111. [CrossRef]
20. Riley, M.R.; Rhiel, M.; Zhou, X.; Arnold, M.A.; Murhammer, D.W. Simultaneous measurement of glucose and glutamine in insect cell culture media by near infrared spectroscopy. *Biotechnol. Bioeng.* **1997**, *55*, 11–15. [CrossRef]
21. Marison, I.W.; Hennessy, S.; Foley, R.; Schuler, M.; Sivaprakasam, S.; Freeland, B. The Choice of Suitable Online Analytical Techniques and Data Processing for Monitoring of Bioprocesses. *Process Integr. Biochem. Eng.* **2012**, *132*, 249–280. [CrossRef]
22. Mercier, S.M.; Rouel, P.M.; Lebrun, P.; Diepenbroek, B.; Wijffels, R.H.; Streefland, M. Process analytical technology tools for perfusion cell culture. *Eng. Life Sci.* **2015**, *16*, 25–35. [CrossRef]
23. Moore, B.; Sanford, R.; Zhang, A. Case study: The characterization and implementation of dielectric spectroscopy (biocapacitance) for process control in a commercial GMP CHO manufacturing process. *Biotechnol. Prog.* **2019**, *35*, e2782. [CrossRef] [PubMed]
24. Opel, C.; Li, J.; Amanullah, A. Quantitative modeling of viable cell density, cell size, intracellular conductivity, and membrane capacitance in batch and fed-batch CHO processes using dielectric spectroscopy. *Biotechnol. Prog.* **2010**, *26*, 1187–1199. [CrossRef] [PubMed]
25. Justice, C.; Brix, A.; Freimark, D.; Kraume, M.; Pfromm, P.; Eichenmueller, B.; Czermak, P. Process control in cell culture technology using dielectric spectroscopy. *Biotechnol. Adv.* **2011**, *29*, 391–401. [CrossRef] [PubMed]
26. Tibayrenc, P.; Preziosi-Belloy, L.; Ghommidh, C. On-line monitoring of dielectrical properties of yeast cells during a stress-model alcoholic fermentation. *Process. Biochem.* **2011**, *46*, 193–201. [CrossRef]
27. Liu, Y.; Wang, Z.; Li, L.; Cui, X.; Chu, J.; Zhang, S.; Zhuang, Y. On-line monitoring of the aggregate size distribution of Carthamus tinctorius L. cells with multi-frequency capacitance measurements. *RSC Adv.* **2016**, *6*, 89764–89769. [CrossRef]
28. Zeiser, A.; Voyer, R.; Jardin, B.; Tom, R.; Kamen, A. On-line monitoring of the progress of infection in Sf-9 insect cell cultures using relative permittivity measurements. *Biotechnol. Bioeng.* **1999**, *63*, 122–126. [CrossRef]
29. Zeiser, A.; Elias, C.; Voyer, R.; Jardin, B.; Kamen, A. On-Line Monitoring of Physiological Parameters of Insect Cell Cultures during the Growth and Infection Process. *Biotechnol. Prog.* **2000**, *16*, 803–808. [CrossRef]
30. Elias, C.B.; Zeiser, A.; Bedard, C.; Kamen, A.A. Enhanced growth of Sf-9 cells to a maximum density of 5.2×10^7 cells per mL and production of β-galactosidase at high cell density by fed batch culture. *Biotechnol. Bioeng.* **2000**, *68*, 381–388. [CrossRef]
31. Negrete, A.; Esteban, G.; Kotin, R.M. Process optimization of large-scale production of recombinant adeno-associated vectors using dielectric spectroscopy. *Appl. Microbiol. Biotechnol.* **2007**, *76*, 761–772. [CrossRef]
32. Ansorge, S.; Esteban, G.; Schmid, G. On-line monitoring of infected Sf-9 insect cell cultures by scanning permittivity measurements and comparison with off-line biovolume measurements. *Cytotechnology* **2007**, *55*, 115–124. [CrossRef]
33. Petiot, E.; Ansorge, S.; Rosa-Calatrava, M.; Kamen, A. Critical phases of viral production processes monitored by capacitance. *J. Biotechnol.* **2017**, *242*, 19–29. [CrossRef] [PubMed]
34. Druzinec, D.; Salzig, D.; Brix, A.; Kraume, M.; Vilcinskas, A.; Kollewe, C.; Czermak, P. Optimization of Insect Cell Based Protein Production Processes—Online Monitoring, Expression Systems, Scale Up. *Process Integr. Biochem. Eng.* **2013**, *136*, 65–100. [CrossRef]
35. Emma, P.; Kamen, A. Real-time monitoring of influenza virus production kinetics in HEK293 cell cultures. *Biotechnol. Prog.* **2012**, *29*, 275–284. [CrossRef] [PubMed]
36. Ansorge, S.; Lanthier, S.; Transfiguracion, J.; Henry, O.; Kamen, A. Monitoring lentiviral vector production kinetics using online permittivity measurements. *Biochem. Eng. J.* **2011**, *54*, 16–25. [CrossRef]
37. Wasilko, D.J.; Lee, S.E.; Stutzman-Engwall, K.J.; Reitz, B.A.; Emmons, T.L.; Mathis, K.J.; Bienkowski, M.J.; Tomaselli, A.G.; Fischer, H.D. The titerless infected-cells preservation and scale-up (TIPS) method for large-scale production of NO-sensitive human soluble guanylate cyclase (sGC) from insect cells infected with recombinant baculovirus. *Protein Expr. Purif.* **2009**, *65*, 122–132. [CrossRef]
38. Kroll, P.; Stelzer, I.V.; Herwig, C. Soft sensor for monitoring biomass subpopulations in mammalian cell culture processes. *Biotechnol. Lett.* **2017**, *39*, 1667–1673. [CrossRef]

39. Dabros, M.; Dennewald, D.; Currie, D.J.; Lee, M.H.; Todd, R.W.; Marison, I.W.; Von Stockar, U. Cole-Cole, linear and multivariate modeling of capacitance data for on-line monitoring of biomass. *Bioprocess Biosyst. Eng.* **2008**, *32*, 161–173. [CrossRef]
40. Bernal, V.; Carinhas, N.; Yokomizo, A.Y.; Carrondo, M.J.; Alves, P.C. Cell density effect in the baculovirus-insect cells system: A quantitative analysis of energetic metabolism. *Biotechnol. Bioeng.* **2009**, *104*, 162–180. [CrossRef]
41. Ferreira, T.B.; Perdigão, R.; Silva, A.C.; Zhang, C.; Auniņš, J.G.; Carrondo, M.J.; Alves, P.C. 293 cell cycle synchronisation adenovirus vector production. *Biotechnol. Prog.* **2009**, *25*, 235–243. [CrossRef]
42. Merten, O.W. AAV vector production: State of the art developments and remaining challenges. *Cell Gene Ther. Insights* **2016**, *2*, 521–551. [CrossRef]
43. Laasfeld, T.; Kopanchuk, S.; Rinken, A. Image-based cell-size estimation for baculovirus quantification. *Biotechniques* **2017**, *63*, 161–168. [CrossRef] [PubMed]
44. Janakiraman, V.; Forrest, W.F.; Chow, B.; Seshagiri, S. A rapid method for estimation of baculovirus titer based on viable cell size. *J. Virol. Methods* **2006**, *132*, 48–58. [CrossRef] [PubMed]

Publisher's Note: MDPI stays neutral with regard to jurisdictional claims in published maps and institutional affiliations.

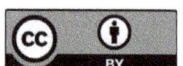

© 2020 by the authors. Licensee MDPI, Basel, Switzerland. This article is an open access article distributed under the terms and conditions of the Creative Commons Attribution (CC BY) license (http://creativecommons.org/licenses/by/4.0/).

MDPI
St. Alban-Anlage 66
4052 Basel
Switzerland
Tel. +41 61 683 77 34
Fax +41 61 302 89 18
www.mdpi.com

Processes Editorial Office
E-mail: processes@mdpi.com
www.mdpi.com/journal/processes